New Insights in the Diagnosis and Treatment of Head and Neck Cancer

Edited by Georgios Giourgos

Published in London, United Kingdom

New Insights in the Diagnosis and Treatment of Head and Neck Cancer
http://dx.doi.org/10.5772/intechopen.1008054
Edited by Georgios Giourgos

Contributors
Abiramasundari V, Alexandra Maria Marin, Alice L. Tang, Amr Allam, Andrea Alberti, Anu Babu, Bianca-Petra Taher, Chad A. Zender, Dustin A. Silverman, Ghazala K. Roshan, Gloria-Simona Bertesteanu, Jay P. Sahu, Jun Zhang, Liam D. Hyland, Mallory McKeon, Megha Mohanakrishnan, Mihai-Dumitru Tudosie, Priscilla F.A. Pichardo, Raluca Grigore, Rohan Thomas Mathew, Rohith R. Menon, Serban Vifor Gabriel Bertesteanu, Shwetima Chaudhary, Simona-Andreea Rujan, Trinanjan Basu, Vishwadeep Mishra

First published in London, United Kingdom, 2026 by IntechOpen
IntechOpen is the global imprint of INTECHOPEN LIMITED, registered in England and Wales, registration number: 11086078, 167-169 Great Portland Street, London, W1W 5PF, United Kingdom

For EU product safety concerns: IN TECH d.o.o., Prolaz Marije Krucifikse Kozulić 3, 51000 Rijeka, Croatia, info@intechopen.com or visit our website at intechopen.com.

British Library Cataloguing-in-Publication Data
A catalogue record for this book is available from the British Library

New Insights in the Diagnosis and Treatment of Head and Neck Cancer
Edited by Georgios Giourgos
p. cm.

This title is part of the Oncology Book Series, Volume 17
Series Editor: Thomas J. FitzGerald
Topic: Cancer Diagnostics and Treatment
Topic Editor: Michael Gibson

Print ISBN 978-1-83635-662-2
Online ISBN 978-1-83635-661-5
eBook (PDF) ISBN 978-1-83635-663-9
ISSN 3049-8864

If disposing of this product, please recycle the paper responsibly.

IntechOpen Book Series
Oncology
Volume 17

Aims and Scope of the Series

The field of oncology has undergone extraordinary change and progress over the past several decades. Today, information is evolving at a rapid rate, with standards of management far different than standards of care applied during the training of most practicing oncologists. Oncology practitioners in all disciplines must remain current to optimize patient care. Basic and translational science remain critical in developing process improvements for patient care. The closer we understand the mechanism, the more we can improve targeted therapies and apply them to patient care. The pace of information is moving faster than at any previous time in history, and all oncology disciplines must remain current to provide excellent service to patients. The modern oncologist must be fluent in using big data and the volume of information generated in clinical trials. As we move closer to personalized patient care based on genomics and molecular biomarkers, the modern oncologist has to be nimble in assessing all available information and how this would be applied to each patient, balanced by the clinical status and medical co-morbidities of each patient. Targeted therapies can bring new and different sequelae, and oncology teams need to remain fluent in managing the consequences of therapy and primary management. In this book series, we will present how modern care has progressed in multiple disease areas and how modern oncology teams need to adapt in order to manage the cancer patients of today successfully. Surgery, radiation therapy, and medical oncology are practiced today with the support of exceptional modern technology, and in this series, we will review how these improvements are applied to each disease site to maintain excellence in patient care.

Meet the Series Editor

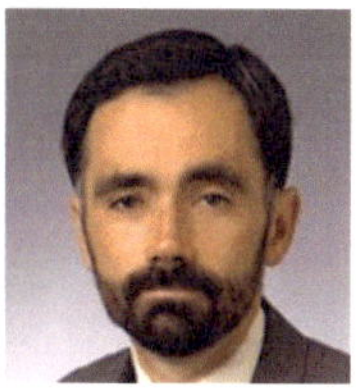

Dr. FitzGerald is the professor and chair of the Department of Radiation Oncology at UMass Chan Medical School in the USA. He serves as one of the principal investigators of the Imaging and Radiation Oncology Core (IROC) service for the National Cancer Institute clinical trials program and is directly involved in the quality assurance of clinical trials in the National Clinical Trials Network (NCTN). Dr. Fitzgerald manages NCTN clinical trials with a real-time pre-therapy review of imaging and radiation therapy treatment objects to ensure the care plan complies with study objectives and the patient stage has been assigned to the correct study. His basic science interest is in hematopoietic stem cell biology and cellular adhesion molecules as they pertain to therapeutic resistance and mitigation of injury from therapy.

Meet the Volume Editor

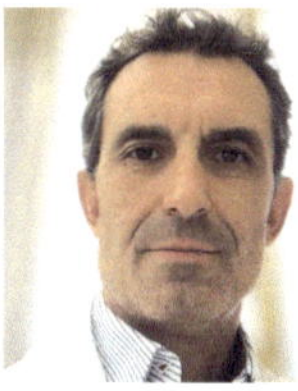

Georgios Giourgos, MD, Ph.D., is a specialist in Otorhinolaryngology-Head and Neck Surgery at the ORL Unit of ASST "Papa Giovanni XXIII" in Bergamo, holding a High Specialization position since 2022. He graduated in Medicine and Surgery with top marks in 2003, completed his ENT specialization with honors in 2009, and earned a Ph.D. in Experimental Surgery and Microsurgery in 2012. With over 2,400 surgical procedures performed, including more than 1,800 as the lead surgeon, he focuses on skull base, head and neck oncology, and paranasal sinus disorders. He has authored numerous scientific publications and is an active member of international scientific societies. He frequently participates in conferences and training courses as a lecturer and invited speaker.

Contents

Preface

Head and neck cancer represents one of the most complex and challenging fields in modern medicine, requiring a multidisciplinary approach that integrates surgical expertise, oncological innovation, advanced radiotherapy techniques, and increasingly precise diagnostic strategies. Continuous scientific progress has profoundly transformed the management of these diseases, leading to improved survival rates, enhanced functional outcomes, and a better quality of life for patients.

New Insights in the Diagnosis and Treatment of Head and Neck Cancer was conceived to provide clinicians, surgeons, oncologists, radiation oncologists, and researchers with an updated overview of the most relevant advances in this rapidly evolving field. The chapters included in this volume explore innovative perspectives in diagnosis and treatment, highlighting both established approaches and emerging strategies that are reshaping contemporary head and neck oncology.

Particular attention has been dedicated to recent developments in minimally invasive and reconstructive surgery, precision radiotherapy, systemic therapies, immunotherapy, and molecular oncology. Furthermore, the book emphasizes the growing importance of personalized medicine, multidisciplinary decision-making, and integrated patient-centered care. Advances in imaging, pathology, and biomolecular research are also discussed, reflecting the crucial role of early diagnosis and tailored therapeutic planning in achieving optimal outcomes.

The management of head and neck malignancies demands close collaboration among specialists from different disciplines. For this reason, this book aims not only to present scientific and technical innovations but also to foster a broader, multidisciplinary perspective that can support daily clinical practice and stimulate further research.

We hope that this volume will serve as a valuable resource for all healthcare professionals involved in the treatment of head and neck cancer, from experienced specialists to young physicians approaching this challenging field. By sharing current knowledge and novel insights, we aspire to contribute to the continuous improvement of patient care and to inspire future developments in head and neck oncology.

Georgios Giourgos, MD, PhD
Otorhinolaryngology Clinic,
ASST "Papa Giovanni XXIII",
Bergamo, Italy

Section 1

Diagnostic Updates

Chapter 1

Optical Coherence Tomography for Early Detection of Nasopharyngeal and Oral Cancers: Technical Advances and Clinical Potential

Jun Zhang

Abstract

Early detection of oral squamous cell carcinoma (OSCC) and nasopharyngeal carcinoma (NPC) continues to present significant clinical challenges. Optical coherence tomography (OCT) offers real-time, micrometer-scale resolution imaging of mucosal microarchitecture, positioning it as a promising adjunct between conventional endoscopy and histopathological analysis. This review synthesizes recent technological advancements—including swept-source OCT, spectral-domain OCT, miniaturized side-viewing probes, and functional modalities such as OCT angiography—and examines the emerging clinical evidence supporting their application in OSCC and NPC. In the oral cavity, OCT has demonstrated diagnostic sensitivity and specificity exceeding 90% in distinguishing high-grade dysplasia from invasive carcinoma. Ex vivo investigations of NPC have similarly reported sensitivities of 90% and specificities of 100%. Concurrently, deep learning algorithms now facilitate automated epithelial segmentation, quantitative biomarker extraction, and progression-free survival prediction, with reported area under the curve (AUC) values reaching 0.886. Despite these advancements, key barriers to broader clinical implementation persist, including limited annotated datasets, inter-device variability, and the paucity of large, multicenter validation trials—particularly in the context of NPC. Looking forward, future research will likely focus on AI-integrated, point-of-care OCT systems and the development of multimodal diagnostic pathways that pair sensitive Epstein–Barr virus (EBV) assays with OCT as a confirmatory tool in high-risk populations.

Keywords: optical coherence tomography (OCT), nasopharyngeal carcinoma, oral cancer, noninvasive imaging, head and neck cancer, early cancer detection

1. Introduction

1.1 The global burden of oral and nasopharyngeal cancers

Head and neck cancers, particularly head and neck squamous cell carcinomas (HNSCCs), continue to represent a significant global health burden. Each year, over

IntechOpen

890,000 new cases are diagnosed, and more than 450,000 deaths are recorded worldwide [1]. Among these, oral squamous cell carcinoma (OSCC) and nasopharyngeal carcinoma (NPC) are among the most prevalent subtypes, with marked geographic disparities. OSCC affects more than 275,000 individuals annually and accounts for a disproportionate number of deaths globally, particularly in developing regions and populations with high exposure to risk factors such as tobacco, betel nut, and alcohol consumption [2]. NPC demonstrates significant regional and ethnic clustering. Incidence rates of 25–50 cases per 100,000 have been reported in Southern China (notably in Guangdong and Guangxi), Southeast Asia, and parts of North Africa [3]. In these regions, NPC is often the most prevalent head and neck malignancy among males under the age of 50. The disease has well-established associations with Epstein–Barr virus (EBV) infection, host genetic susceptibility (e.g., HLA genotypes), and dietary exposure to nitrosamines [3].

Despite improvements in treatment access, both OSCC and NPC are frequently diagnosed at advanced stages. Approximately 50% of OSCC cases are identified at stage III or IV, where the five-year survival rate declines to 30–50%. In contrast, early-stage diagnosis (stage I or II) is associated with survival rates exceeding 90% [4]. Similarly, over 85% of NPC patients present with cervical lymph node involvement or distant metastasis at the time of diagnosis [5]. These statistics underscore the critical importance of early detection in improving clinical outcomes, preserving function, and reducing disease-specific mortality. Nevertheless, existing diagnostic and screening frameworks often fail to provide adequate sensitivity or scalability, particularly in high-risk and resource-limited environments.

1.2 Limitations of current diagnostic modalities

Conventional diagnostic practice continues to rely heavily on clinical examination and confirmatory tissue biopsy. While these remain the standard of care, they are not without limitations. OSCC frequently arises from oral potentially malignant disorders (OPMDs), such as leukoplakia, erythroplakia, and oral submucous fibrosis. These precursor lesions often exhibit nonspecific or subtle clinical features, complicating timely recognition. Furthermore, progression from OPMDs to carcinoma may occur over an extended period, necessitating long-term surveillance. In many cases, biopsy is triggered only by overt clinical signs, such as ulceration or induration, leading to delays in diagnosis. Accessibility challenges and subjectivity in clinical judgment further exacerbate diagnostic inefficiencies.

Even when a biopsy is performed, sampling error remains a concern, particularly when lesions are multifocal or located in anatomically complex regions such as the posterior tongue, floor of the mouth, or soft palate [6].

Diagnosing NPC presents even greater challenges due to its deep-seated anatomical location. The nasopharynx is situated posterior to the nasal cavity and superior to the oropharynx, rendering it inaccessible to routine visual inspection. Although nasoendoscopy facilitates direct visualization, it remains limited in detecting subepithelial alterations [7]. Biopsy in this region often requires specialized expertise and anesthesia, making it less feasible in low-resource settings.

Adjunctive diagnostic tools—such as toluidine blue staining, autofluorescence imaging (AFI), narrow-band imaging (NBI), and brush cytology—can enhance visual assessment but are often hindered by variable sensitivity and specificity. For instance, AFI tends to produce high false-positive rates due to its responsiveness to inflammation, which may lead to unnecessary biopsies and elevated patient anxiety [8].

Moreover, there is a lack of diagnostic continuity across different levels of care. Primary care providers, especially in rural or underserved settings, frequently lack access to advanced diagnostic modalities such as histopathology, further contributing to late-stage presentations.

1.3 The rise of optical coherence tomography in oncology

Optical coherence tomography (OCT) has emerged as a promising imaging modality capable of addressing many of the aforementioned limitations. OCT offers real-time, non-invasive, cross-sectional visualization of tissue architecture using low-coherence interferometry. With imaging depths of 1.5 to 2 mm and micrometer-level resolution, OCT is particularly well-suited to assess mucosal surfaces and detect early neoplastic changes [9].

Originally developed for ophthalmologic applications, OCT has been increasingly adapted for oncologic use over the past decade. In oral cancer imaging, OCT enables the evaluation of:

- Epithelial thickness and organization,
- Disruption of natural stratification,
- Discontinuities in the basement membrane,
- Alterations in subepithelial microarchitecture.

These features demonstrate strong correlation with histopathologic markers of moderate-to-severe dysplasia and invasive carcinoma [10, 11].

For nasopharyngeal applications, catheter-based full-range Fourier-domain OCT systems have been developed to navigate the upper airway. One such system, described in studies [12], incorporates a 1.2 mm diameter probe with a 20 mm working range, allowing efficient imaging of the nasal cavity, nasopharynx, and larynx within 40 seconds.

Clinical trials continue to affirm the diagnostic value of OCT. For instance, James et al. demonstrated that spectral-domain OCT (SD-OCT) achieved a sensitivity of 95% and specificity of 76% for identifying oral dysplasia, with sensitivity and specificity values of 93 and 74%, respectively, for distinguishing OSCC from non-malignant tissue [13].

1.4 Clinical rationale and scope of this review

Although research into the use of OCT for cancer diagnostics has progressed significantly, existing reviews often remain narrowly scoped—focusing on specific anatomical targets, isolated OCT technologies, or single-use scenarios such as surgical margin evaluation. A broader synthesis is therefore needed to consolidate current technical advances with emerging clinical insights.

This review aims to bridge that gap by providing an integrated perspective on:

- Recent innovations in OCT system design and catheter development;
- Accumulating empirical evidence supporting OCT's diagnostic potential in OSCC and NPC;

- The growing role of artificial intelligence in image interpretation and classification;
- The challenges and possibilities of incorporating OCT into clinical workflows.

Rather than positioning OCT as a fully established clinical tool, this review highlights its promising potential in facilitating earlier detection and non-invasive evaluation—particularly in high-risk populations and anatomically challenging regions. The goal is to inform future clinical translation and guide ongoing technical refinement.

2. Technological foundations of optical coherence tomography (OCT)

2.1 Physical principles of optical coherence tomography

Optical coherence tomography (OCT) is a non-invasive, light-based imaging modality that enables high-resolution visualization of biological tissues. The technique is grounded in low-coherence interferometry, whereby the time delay and intensity of backscattered light are measured to construct cross-sectional images of tissue microarchitecture. Functionally analogous to ultrasound imaging, OCT achieves significantly higher spatial resolution—typically 2–15 μm axially and 10–50 μm laterally—by utilizing light rather than acoustic waves [9].

A principal advantage of OCT in oncologic applications lies in its capacity to delineate epithelial and stromal layers with high fidelity. These layers are critical for the detection of early neoplastic alterations, particularly in mucosal tissues such as the oral cavity and nasopharynx. OCT's penetration depth of approximately 1.5 to 2 mm in soft tissue is sufficient to resolve microstructural changes that are often indicative of early malignancy [9, 13].

2.2 System design and architecture

All OCT systems operate on the principle of comparing light reflected from the tissue of interest with light reflected from a reference mirror. The fundamental components of an OCT system include the following:

- A broadband light source (e.g., superluminescent diode or swept-source laser),
- A fiber-optic interferometer (commonly of the Michelson type),
- A scanning unit (incorporating galvo mirrors, MEMS actuators, or rotary motors),
- A detection system (spectrometer or photodiode), and
- A signal acquisition and image reconstruction platform.

Two primary system architectures are widely employed: spectral-domain OCT (SD-OCT) and swept-source OCT (SS-OCT). In SD-OCT, the interference spectrum is captured via a spectrometer, while SS-OCT utilizes a tunable laser source that sweeps through a range of wavelengths, with detection by a single photodiode. SS-OCT offers advantages in imaging depth, reduced signal degradation with depth (sensitivity roll-off), and faster acquisition speeds, making it particularly advantageous for assessing anatomically complex regions such as the oral cavity and nasopharynx [14, 15].

2.3 Evolution of OCT modalities

2.3.1 Time-domain OCT (TD-OCT)

TD-OCT represents the first generation of OCT technology, wherein depth-resolved imaging was achieved by mechanically translating the reference mirror. Although foundational, TD-OCT was limited by low acquisition speed (~400 A-scans per second) and vulnerability to motion artifacts, rendering it largely obsolete for contemporary clinical applications [16].

2.3.2 Spectral-domain OCT (SD-OCT)

SD-OCT marked a significant advancement by eliminating mechanical scanning in the reference arm. Instead, it captures the interference spectrum through a stationary spectrometer, enabling acquisition rates up to 250,000 A-scans per second [17]. This enhanced speed and resolution make SD-OCT particularly suitable for dynamic anatomical regions, such as the tongue or vocal cords, and effective in detecting pathologies including epithelial hyperplasia, dysplasia, and early-stage carcinoma (**Figure 1**).

2.3.3 Swept-source OCT (SS-OCT)

SS-OCT replaces the broadband light source with a wavelength-tunable laser that scans through a defined spectral range. This configuration reduces sensitivity roll-off and extends imaging depth (>3 mm), enabling comprehensive evaluation of deeper epithelial and stromal tissues. Additionally, the compact and flexible design of SS-OCT systems supports catheter-based imaging, which is advantageous for nasopharyngeal applications (**Figure 2**) [18].

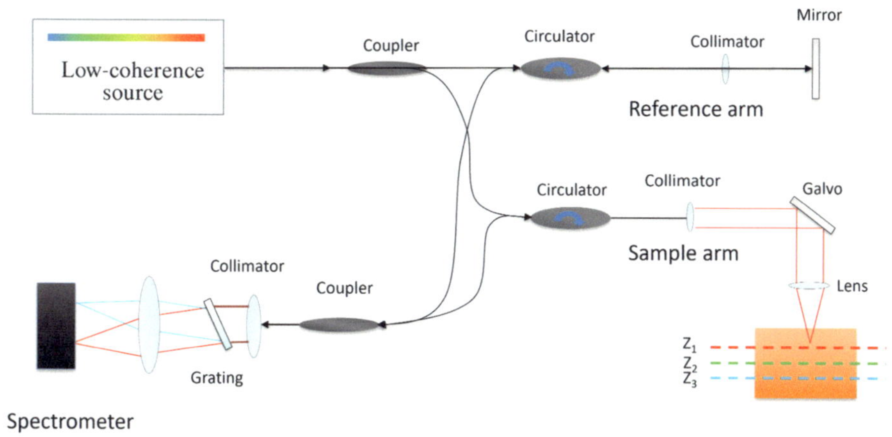

Figure 1.
Schematic of a spectral-domain OCT system employing a broadband light source and spectrometer-based detection.

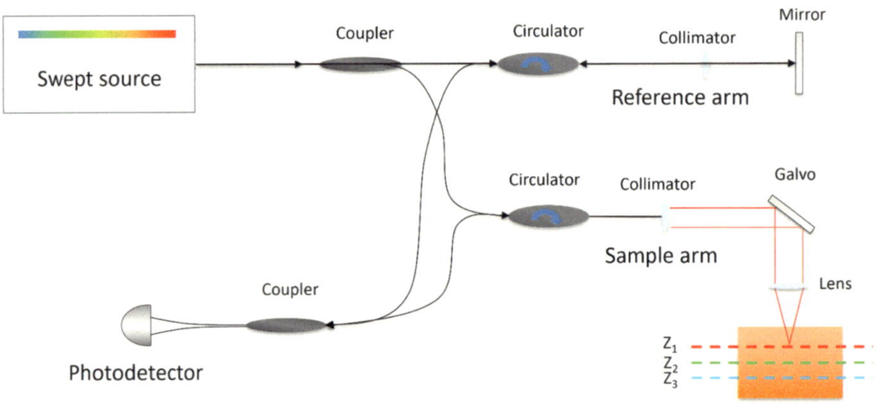

Figure 2.
Schematic of a swept-source optical coherence tomography (SS-OCT) system using a wavelength-swept source and interferometric detection.

2.4 Functional OCT variants and enhancements

2.4.1 Polarization-sensitive OCT (PS-OCT)

PS-OCT extends traditional OCT by detecting changes in light polarization, which arise from tissue birefringence. This capability allows for functional imaging of tissues with varying molecular organization, such as collagen-rich stroma and keratinized epithelium. In the context of oral imaging—where thick keratin layers (e.g., on the tongue dorsum or hard palate) can obscure conventional OCT signals—PS-OCT provides complementary contrast. While promising for identifying early microstructural and birefringence abnormalities, its specificity in distinguishing benign from dysplastic or malignant keratinized tissue remains under active investigation [19].

2.4.2 Doppler OCT and optical microangiography (OMAG)

Doppler OCT and OMAG leverage phase or frequency shifts in backscattered light caused by moving blood cells to generate vascular imaging. These techniques enable the visualization of microcirculatory changes, including vessel density, flow velocity, and perfusion heterogeneity—parameters often altered in neoplastic progression [20]. OMAG, or OCT angiography (OCTA), offers label-free, depth-resolved imaging of capillary networks, allowing early detection of tumor-associated angiogenesis with high spatial resolution [21].

2.5 Miniaturization and endoscopic integration

To facilitate imaging in anatomically restricted regions such as the nasopharynx, miniaturized OCT probes have been developed. Jing et al. reported a 1.2 mm diameter endoscopic probe integrated with a rotational scanning catheter capable of capturing high-resolution images of the upper airway in under 40 seconds [12]. Further innovations include real-time anatomical tracking algorithms and motion stabilization software, which enhance imaging reliability during dynamic physiological conditions such as respiration (**Figure 3**) [22, 23].

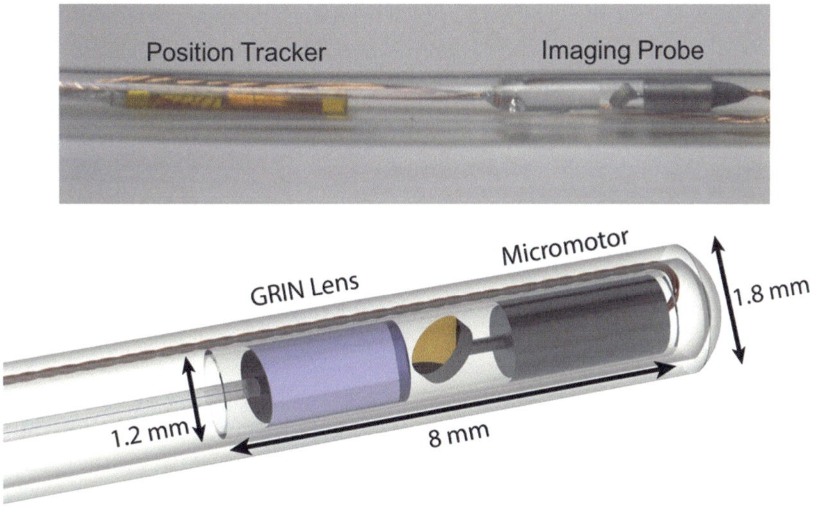

Figure 3.
Fully integrated side-viewing OCT imaging probe with positional tracking capabilities optimized for nasopharyngeal imaging. (Top) Photograph of the integrated probe, showing the micromotor-driven imaging unit and electromagnetic position tracker. (Bottom) Schematic rendering of the optical assembly, featuring a GRIN lens, 45° micromirror, and high-speed micromotor enclosed in a 1.2 mm outer diameter capillary. This compact design enables access to anatomically constrained regions such as the nasal cavity and nasopharynx. Adapted from Jing et al., Scientific Reports 2023, under Creative Commons Attribution License [22].

2.6 Summary and outlook

The technological evolution of OCT has progressed from early, mechanically constrained systems to advanced, high-speed imaging platforms capable of resolving fine tissue structures in complex anatomical sites. Key innovations—such as swept-source lasers, miniaturized endoscopic probes, and functional imaging variants like OCT angiography and PS-OCT—have broadened its applicability in oncologic diagnostics.

These technological foundations set the stage for expanding OCT into clinical applications. The following sections explore its role in oral and nasopharyngeal cancer imaging, including lesion surveillance and intraoperative assessment. The integration of artificial intelligence for image interpretation is addressed in Section 5.

3. Optical coherence tomography in oral cancer imaging

3.1 Clinical relevance and imaging needs

The clinical prognosis of oral squamous cell carcinoma (OSCC) is strongly correlated with the stage at diagnosis. Early-stage OSCC (stages I–II) is associated with markedly improved survival rates and better preservation of oral function compared to advanced disease [24]. However, early lesions frequently present with subtle or nonspecific clinical features, leading to delayed recognition and diagnosis. In most cases, definitive diagnosis is only achieved through biopsy following the development of overt symptoms [25].

Oral potentially malignant disorders (OPMDs), such as leukoplakia, erythroplakia, oral lichen planus (OLP), and oral submucous fibrosis (OSMF), serve as established precursor conditions for OSCC. The risk of malignant transformation among these entities varies significantly based on both clinical presentation and histopathological criteria [26]. Nevertheless, visual assessment alone often proves insufficient, particularly in anatomically complex or less accessible regions such as the posterior tongue, retromolar area, and floor of the mouth [25]. These factors contribute to under-diagnosis and inconsistent follow-up, limiting opportunities for timely intervention.

Although histopathological biopsy remains the gold standard for diagnosing epithelial dysplasia and early invasive disease, it presents several limitations. The invasive nature of the procedure, combined with sampling error and prolonged turnaround times, can hinder timely and accurate clinical decision-making. Moreover, in cases involving multifocal lesions or widespread mucosal changes, repeated biopsies are often impractical or poorly tolerated.

In this context, optical coherence tomography (OCT) offers a promising adjunctive imaging modality capable of addressing several diagnostic limitations. By providing real-time, high-resolution cross-sectional images of the epithelial and subepithelial layers, OCT facilitates non-invasive evaluation of mucosal microarchitecture. Its micrometer-level axial resolution allows clinicians to detect early neoplastic changes and monitor OPMDs longitudinally, thereby improving diagnostic confidence and potentially reducing the need for repeat or unnecessary biopsies in selected clinical contexts [27].

3.2 Optical hallmarks of OSCC and OPMDs in OCT imaging

OCT enables the identification of specific microarchitectural alterations that distinguish between normal oral mucosa, OPMDs, and invasive squamous cell carcinoma. These diagnostic features are primarily based on variations in epithelial thickness, structural organization, basement membrane continuity, and subepithelial reflectivity patterns (**Table 1**) [28].

These imaging characteristics demonstrate strong concordance with histopathologic criteria, allowing clinicians to non-invasively stratify lesion severity during examination. For instance, Sunny et al. reported that SD-OCT imaging achieved over 90% concordance with histological grading when assessing epithelial architecture in oral lesions [29]. Such findings underscore the utility of OCT in augmenting clinical decision-making, particularly for early-stage disease and longitudinal surveillance of OPMDs. By offering a real-time, tissue-preserving alternative to biopsy, OCT enhances the diagnostic workflow and supports timely identification of high-risk lesions.

Tissue Condition	Representative OCT Features
Normal mucosa	Well-organized stratified epithelium with homogenous reflectivity; intact, continuous basement membrane
Mild dysplasia	Mild epithelial thickening; partial loss of normal stratification; basement membrane remains continuous
Moderate-to-severe dysplasia	Disruption of epithelial stratification; increased optical heterogeneity; basement membrane appears fragmented or indistinct
Invasive carcinoma	Complete epithelial disarray; absence of discernible basement membrane; stromal disorganization and irregular scattering

Table 1.
Representative OCT imaging features for oral mucosal conditions.

Study (year)	OCT modality	Sensitivity	Specificity	Sample size
Wilder-Smith et al. [10]	SD-OCT	≈93%	≈93–97%	50 lesions
Yang et al. [30]	SS-OCT	97.9%	83.8%	14 samples
Meta-analysis, 2024	SD-/SS-/PS-/AI-enhanced OCT	75–100%	71–100%	860 events (cancer detections)
Jerjes et al. [31]	Multi-beam OCT	>80%	>80%	120 patients

Table 2.
Summary of reported diagnostic performance of OCT modalities for oral cancer detection.

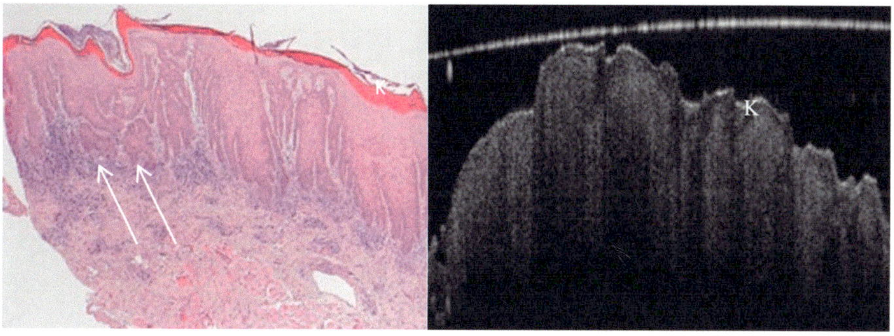

Figure 4.
Comparison of OCT and histopathology in severe dysplasia. Representative cross-sectional OCT image (right) and corresponding hematoxylin–eosin (H&E) section (left) of speckled leukoplakia from the floor of the mouth, demonstrating epithelial thickening, keratinization (K), and disruption of epithelial stratification. Adapted from Jerjes et al., Journal of Clinical Medicine 2024, under Creative Commons Attribution License [30].

3.3 Clinical studies on OCT in oral cancer detection

A growing body of clinical evidence supports the diagnostic utility of OCT in detecting OSCC and OPMDs. Studies employing various OCT modalities—including SD-OCT, SS-OCT, and systems enhanced with artificial intelligence—have consistently demonstrated high sensitivity and specificity in differentiating malignant and premalignant lesions (**Table 2, Figure 4**) [10, 30–32].

In parallel, pilot programs have validated the operational feasibility of deploying portable, low-cost OCT systems in resource-constrained settings. One such initiative in Bangalore, India, successfully integrated a mobile OCT unit into a cancer center's diagnostic workflow. The system maintained strong diagnostic accuracy and demonstrated promise for expansion into community-based screening, particularly in regions with limited access to standard histopathological services [33].

4. Optical coherence tomography in nasopharyngeal cancer imaging

4.1 Clinical importance and diagnostic gaps in nasopharyngeal carcinoma

Nasopharyngeal carcinoma (NPC) is a distinct epithelial malignancy characterized by pronounced ethnic and geographical clustering. In endemic regions—such as Southern China, Southeast Asia, and North Africa—the age-standardized incidence ranges from 25 to 50 per 100,000 individuals, with NPC ranking among the top three malignancies in males under 50 years of age [3].

Despite the implementation of Epstein–Barr virus (EBV)-based serological screening and routine nasoendoscopy, over 80% of NPC cases are still diagnosed at advanced stages (III–IV), often with nodal metastasis or skull base invasion [5]. Early-stage NPC, particularly T1 lesions restricted to the fossa of Rosenmüller, are commonly subclinical and submucosal, posing significant challenges to detection via conventional white-light endoscopy.

Histopathological confirmation through biopsy remains the diagnostic gold standard. However, nasopharyngeal biopsy is invasive and often limited in accessing anatomically recessed areas. These technical limitations contribute to diagnostic delays and under-detection of early disease.

4.2 Anatomical and optical imaging challenges of the nasopharynx

The nasopharynx constitutes a narrow, posteriorly curved anatomical compartment bordered anteriorly by the choanae and posteriorly by the cervical spine.

Key challenges limiting conventional imaging include the following:

- Incomplete visualization of lateral recesses via endoscopy.
- Submucosal tumor growth not apparent on surface inspection.
- Motion artifacts related to breathing and swallowing.
- Mucosal folds and tissue heterogeneity that scatter incident light, degrading optical resolution.

Cross-sectional imaging modalities such as computed tomography (CT) and magnetic resonance imaging (MRI) lack the resolution necessary to detect epithelial-level dysplasia. Although nasoendoscopy offers surface-level visualization, it may fail to detect deeper pathological changes. Moreover, repeated biopsies carry procedural risks and are associated with patient discomfort and increased healthcare burden.

To address the inherent limitations of conventional imaging modalities in the nasopharyngeal region, catheter-based OCT systems have been developed to facilitate high-resolution, long-range imaging of the complex upper airway anatomy. The incorporation of side-viewing probes and extended scanning ranges—reaching up to 30 mm—permits comprehensive, circumferential visualization of the nasopharyngeal cavity, including anatomically challenging regions that are typically inaccessible by standard approaches [22]. When integrated with positional tracking systems, these catheter-based OCT platforms enable spatially registered three-dimensional reconstructions of the upper airway. This capability supports precise anatomical localization and offers the potential for longitudinal assessment and follow-up [15]. Furthermore, advancements in motion-resolved and compliance-sensitive OCT techniques have introduced new opportunities for characterizing nasopharyngeal tissue biomechanics. Notably, localized compliance mapping has been applied in awake human subjects to assess airway collapsibility, thereby contributing valuable insights into functional tissue properties (**Figure 5**) [23].

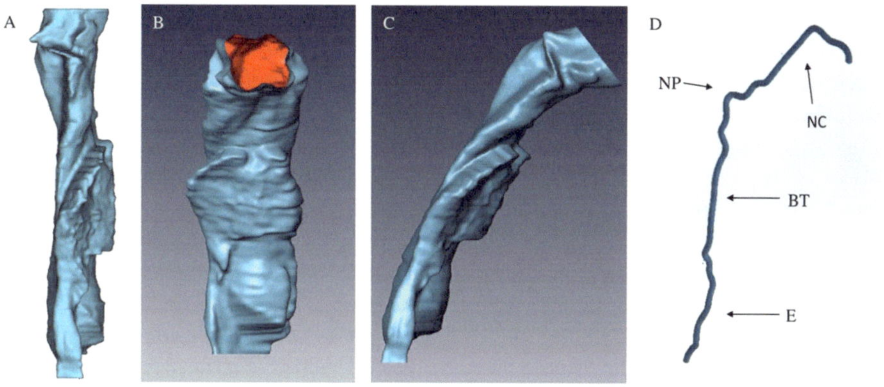

Figure 5.
3D reconstruction of the upper airway using long-range optical coherence tomography (LR-OCT) with integrated position tracking. (A) Model without positional tracking, showing linear stacking of cross-sections with anatomical distortion. (B, C) Anterior and lateral views of anatomically correct reconstructions using real-time probe tracking, allowing accurate localization of regions such as the nasal cavity (NC), nasopharynx (NP), base of tongue (BT), and epiglottis (E). Adapted from Jing et al., Scientific Reports 2023, under Creative Commons Attribution License [22].

4.3 Optical markers of NPC on OCT

Catheter-based Fourier-domain OCT systems provide real-time cross-sectional imaging with axial resolutions of 7–10 μm and tissue penetration depths of up to 2 mm [12, 18, 22]. Both clinical and preclinical studies have identified characteristic optical signatures of early-stage NPC, including:

- Epithelial thickening and architectural disorganization [34].
- Loss of epithelial stratification [35].
- Disruption or blurring of the basement membrane [35].
- Localized high-scattering zones in the submucosa.
- Microvascular alterations—such as neovascularization, increased capillary density or disorganized loops—readily detectable with optical microangiography [21].

These imaging features correlate with moderate-to-severe dysplasia and have been validated against histological findings in both animal models and human studies.

4.4 Clinical studies and pilot trials

Initial ex vivo investigations established that OCT is capable of replicating the laminar architecture of nasopharyngeal mucosa with a diagnostic performance closely approximating that of frozen-section histology. In a pilot study involving ten freshly excised biopsy specimens (five NPC and five normal), Li et al. demonstrated that normal mucosa is characterized by a clearly discernible three-layer configuration: the superficial epithelium, a hyper-reflective basement membrane interface, and the underlying lamina propria. In contrast, NPC samples exhibited a complete loss of this stratification, with basement membrane discontinuity and either hyporeflective or hyperintense irregularities in the submucosal region [35]. Using a diagnostic criterion based on "loss of layer architecture with or without basement membrane breach," the study achieved 90% sensitivity and 100% specificity in distinguishing NPC from normal tissue. These imaging features have since been adopted as reference standards in subsequent feasibility assessments.

To assess translational safety and workflow feasibility, Sun et al. conducted a study using a 1.7 mm-diameter, 1310 nm OCT probe, which was introduced transnasally under topical anesthesia in ten adult subjects. The probe was advanced to the pharyngeal orifice of the eustachian tube. Each examination lasted approximately 3 minutes (mean: 2.8 ± 1.6 minutes), was well tolerated with no adverse events, and generated high-resolution cross-sectional images delineating the lumen, mucosa, submucosa, and cartilage to a depth of approximately 2 mm. These findings confirmed the procedural safety and anatomical accessibility of rigid pull-back OCT imaging within the nasopharyngeal recess—an area critical to NPC screening [36].

Although dedicated clinical trials in NPC remain limited, the broader body of evidence supporting intraoperative OCT in head and neck oncology is growing. A 2022 systematic review published in Cancers (MDPI) synthesized findings from 23 intraoperative imaging studies, identifying two that employed OCT—one in laryngeal and one in oral squamous cell carcinoma. Reported diagnostic performance ranged from 76% accuracy in the laryngeal application to 100% sensitivity and specificity in the oral cancer cohort, specifically for surgical margin assessment [37]. Although none of the included studies focused on the nasopharynx, these results underscore OCT's potential as a real-time adjunct to endoscopy and conventional cross-sectional imaging in complex head and neck procedures.

Recent pilot studies have also begun to extend the anatomical scope and functional utility of OCT in upper airway imaging. High-resolution OCT has successfully been used to visualize dynamic physiological processes, including real-time ciliary motion and mucociliary transport, thus demonstrating the modality's applicability beyond static morphological assessment [38]. Additionally, the integration of structural OCT with OCT angiography has enabled visualization and quantification of microvascular networks in vascular skull base lesions—such as glomus jugulare tumors and facial nerve schwannomas. These findings highlight the potential for optical vascular biomarkers to aid in differentiating middle ear and skull base pathologies at the point of care [39].

5. Artificial intelligence and OCT interpretation

5.1 Motivation for AI integration

The interpretation of OCT images, particularly in the context of detecting early-stage malignancies, necessitates sub-cellular level discrimination that can challenge even experienced clinicians and yield variable results. The integration of artificial intelligence (AI) into OCT analysis has emerged as a strategy to enhance diagnostic consistency and accuracy.

5.2 AI-driven OCT interpretation for early oral cancer

These AI frameworks generate quantitative parameter maps—such as epithelial thickness, local attenuation coefficients, and texture entropy—which are

Study (year)	AI method/architecture	OCT modality	Performance
Hill et al. [40]	3-D U-Net ensemble, epithelial surface & E-S boundary masks	SS-OCT (endoscopic oral)	Dice 0.98 (surface) / 0.83 (E-S); better than 5 expert raters (0.95–0.97 / 0.64–0.78)
Malone et al. [42]	U-Net segmentation, 7 quantitative biomarkers	Wide-field SS-OCT (oral cavity) – dysplasia vs. carcinoma	Lesion vs. contralateral: epi-depth, E–S boundary loss, epi-attenuation (all $p < 0.05$)
Yuan et al. [41]	Multi-view deep-radiomics (MC3 CNN features + blood immune indices)	Ultra-HR SD-OCT (ex-vivo oral specimens) – prognostic model (PFS)	AUC 0.886 for progression-free survival prediction

Table 3.
Representative studies integrating AI with OCT for early detection of oral cancer [40–42].

subsequently incorporated into risk stratification models or logistic regression-based prognostic classifiers (**Table 3**).

Key clinical insights include the following:

- *Diagnostic accuracy:* As summarized in the systematic review by Jerjes et al. [30, 32], single-center studies consistently report that AI-assisted OCT systems achieve sensitivity or specificity values exceeding 90% for the differentiation of moderate-to-severe dysplasia from invasive carcinoma within the oral cavity.

- *Segmentation-driven pipelines:* Hill et al. implemented a 3-D U-Net ensemble to generate voxel-wise segmentation masks of both the epithelial surface and the epithelial–stromal interface. These masks were then transformed into en-face maps quantifying epithelial thickness and stratification, which served as the basis for downstream feature extraction and longitudinal lesion monitoring [40]. Complementarily, Malone et al. demonstrated that a set of seven interpretable structural metrics—encompassing epithelial thickness, optical scattering coefficients, and boundary continuity—could distinguish lesions from contralateral mucosa without requiring a CNN-based classifier [42].

- *Prognostic modeling:* Extending beyond binary classification, Yuan et al. integrated OCT-derived radiomic features with systemic inflammatory biomarkers to predict clinical outcomes. Their model achieved an area under the curve (AUC) of 0.886 for progression-free survival, indicating that OCT texture-based analytics may offer prognostic information complementary to traditional staging systems [41].

Nasopharyngeal Imaging Gap:

At present, the application of AI-enhanced OCT in the nasopharyngeal region remains nascent. Most existing efforts are limited to rule-based segmentation techniques or preliminary transfer-learning experiments with small datasets. This represents a significant opportunity for translational adaptation of established oral-cavity AI pipelines, contingent upon the future availability of large-scale imaging datasets from anatomical sites such as the Eustachian tube and the fossa of Rosenmüller.

6. Challenges and future directions

6.1 Current barriers to clinical integration

Despite significant technical progress, several critical barriers continue to impede the widespread clinical adoption of OCT, particularly within oncological settings:

- Variability in device architecture and imaging parameters across manufacturers compromises cross-study comparability and limits the generalizability of findings.
- The absence of standardized acquisition protocols and annotation frameworks presents substantial challenges for the training and benchmarking of AI models.
- A paucity of high-quality annotated datasets—especially for NPC—hampers the development, validation, and clinical translation of AI-OCT systems.
- Patient-specific anatomical heterogeneity, particularly in regions characterized by deep curvature or mucosal complexity, introduces inconsistencies in image acquisition and interpretation.
- The interpretability of AI outputs remains a pressing concern, underscoring the urgent need for explainable AI methodologics to ensure clinical trustworthiness and facilitate regulatory approval.

A notable discrepancy persists in the maturity of OCT applications between OSCC and NPC. The relative accessibility of oral lesions permits routine scanning with standard handheld probes and supports the generation of large-scale imaging datasets. By contrast, the anatomically constrained nasopharynx necessitates the use of ultra-miniaturized, side-viewing catheter systems capable of long-range scanning—an engineering challenge that, coupled with the limited accessibility of biopsy specimens and the scarcity of annotated training data, continues to delay OCT validation and clinical implementation in NPC contexts [22, 23].

6.2 Future perspectives and emerging directions

OCT is progressively transitioning from proof-of-concept applications to early clinical adoption. Key future directions include the following:

- Catheter and system design optimization: the development of sub-millimeter diameter probes with wide-field, side-viewing optics and high-speed acquisition rates (>200 kHz A-scans/s) is expected to enhance image resolution and coverage in the nasopharyngeal cavity.
- AI-integrated diagnosis: Embedding deep learning algorithms directly into OCT platforms will enable real-time tissue classification and malignancy risk estimation, thereby expanding the utility of OCT in low-resource or point-of-care settings [30–32].
- Telemedicine and mobile health integration: The coupling of portable OCT systems with 5G-enabled cloud platforms offers potential for remote diagnosis and longitudinal monitoring in high-incidence or underserved regions.

- Multimodal screening pathways. Large prospective trials have established plasma-DNA (Chan 2017 [43]) and serology-based (Chen 2025 [44]). EBV assays as effective first-line tools for NPC screening—Chan reported sensitivity 97% and specificity 99%, while Chen's cluster-randomized trial achieved a 30% reduction in NPC mortality. Given OCT's ability to visualize sub-millimeter mucosal change in vivo, adding high-resolution nasopharyngeal OCT as a second-tier confirmatory test could, in principle, further boost specificity and spare low-risk individuals unnecessary biopsy—an hypothesis now ripe for prospective evaluation.

- Intraoperative applications: OCT may provide valuable intraoperative guidance for margin assessment and residual tumor detection during surgical resections of OSCC and NPC.

Collectively, these innovations suggest that OCT may evolve into a versatile platform for early detection, diagnosis, and intraoperative guidance across the cancer care continuum. However, this vision is contingent upon successful validation through multicenter, prospective trials and alignment with international regulatory frameworks.

7. Conclusion

OCT has progressed from a laboratory innovation to a clinically viable imaging modality, offering real-time visualization of sub-millimeter mucosal structures with high fidelity. In the context of oral oncology, handheld and catheter-based spectral-domain and swept-source OCT systems routinely achieve axial resolutions of 5–10 μm, demonstrating diagnostic sensitivities and specificities exceeding 90% in differentiating moderate-to-severe dysplasia from invasive carcinoma. This performance is underpinned by three critical technological advancements: high-speed swept-source lasers that minimize sensitivity roll-off, miniaturized side-viewing probes enabling comprehensive circumferential imaging, and functional extensions such as OCT angiography that delineate tumor-associated microvascular changes.

While nasopharyngeal applications have historically lagged due to anatomical and technical constraints, rapid progress has been made. Catheter-based probes with diameters of $\leq$ 1.7 mm have been safely navigated to the pharyngeal orifice of the eustachian tube in awake individuals, generating laminar imaging comparable to ex vivo frozen-section histology. Preliminary clinical studies validate procedural tolerability and reveal optical hallmarks—epithelial disorganization, basement membrane disruption, and submucosal heterogeneity—that are consistent with established oncologic criteria in the oral cavity.

The integration of AI is accelerating the clinical readiness of OCT. Deep learning architectures, such as U-Net-based 3D segmentation models, now achieve Dice coefficients as high as 0.98 for epithelial boundary detection, often surpassing human expert performance. Additionally, radiomics frameworks that integrate OCT-derived texture features with systemic inflammatory biomarkers have demonstrated prognostic utility, with progression-free survival prediction reaching an AUC of 0.886. These AI pipelines transform qualitative OCT datasets into standardized, reproducible biomarkers amenable to longitudinal tracking and integration into digital health infrastructures, including deployment on portable OCT platforms suitable for low-resource environments.

Nevertheless, several barriers persist. Device heterogeneity, limited availability of annotated datasets—particularly for nasopharyngeal carcinoma—and the absence of large-scale, multicenter validation studies continue to impede regulatory clearance and widespread adoption. Emerging solutions such as explainable AI (XAI) models and federated learning frameworks may address data-sharing limitations, while continued innovations in sub-millimeter catheter fabrication and motion-compensated acquisition protocols remain essential for reliable nasopharyngeal imaging. Furthermore, combining ultrahigh-sensitivity EBV assays with OCT-based secondary triage holds promise for improving diagnostic specificity and reducing unnecessary biopsies—though this strategy remains to be rigorously evaluated.

In conclusion, OCT is uniquely positioned to bridge the diagnostic divide between gross endoscopic assessment and histopathological confirmation in head and neck malignancies. With continued convergence across photonics, catheter engineering, and AI, OCT is poised to evolve from a complementary imaging technique into a central platform for early detection, risk stratification, and intraoperative guidance in both oral and nasopharyngeal cancer care.

Author details

Jun Zhang[1,2]

1 Institute of Ophthalmic Diseases, Guangxi Academy of Medical Sciences, Nanning, Guangxi, China

2 School of Electronics and Information Engineering, Ningbo University of Technology, Ningbo, Zhejiang, China

*Address all correspondence to: junzhang8819@gmail.com

References

[1] Johnson DE, Burtness B, Leemans CR, Lui VW, Bauman JE, Grandis JR. Head and neck squamous cell carcinoma. Nature Reviews Disease Primers. 2020;**6**(1):92. DOI: 10.1038/s41572-023-00418-5

[2] Sung H, Ferlay J, Siegel RL, Laversanne M, Soerjomataram I, Jemal A, et al. Global cancer statistics 2020: GLOBOCAN estimates of incidence and mortality worldwide for 36 cancers in 185 countries. CA: A Cancer Journal for Clinicians. 2021;**71**(3):209-249. DOI: 10.3322/caac.21660

[3] Chang ET, Adami HO. The enigmatic epidemiology of nasopharyngeal carcinoma. Cancer Epidemiology Biomarkers and Prevention. 2006;**15**(10):1765-1777. DOI: 10.1158/1055-9965.EPI-06-0353

[4] Mauceri R, Bazzano M, Coppini M, Tozzo P, Panzarella V, Campisi G. Diagnostic delay of oral squamous cell carcinoma and the fear of diagnosis: A scoping review. Frontiers in Psychology. 2022;**13**:1009080. DOI: 10.3389/fpsyg.2022.1009080

[5] Wang X, Hu C, Ying H, He X, Zhu G, Kong L, et al. Patterns of lymph node metastasis from nasopharyngeal carcinoma based on the 2013 updated consensus guidelines for neck node levels. Radiotherapy and Oncology. 2015;**115**(1):41-45. DOI: 10.1016/j.radonc.2015.02.017

[6] Villa A, Villa C, Abati S. Oral cancer and oral erythroplakia: An update and implication for clinicians. Australian Dental Journal. 2011;**56**(3):253-256. DOI: 10.1111/j.1834-7819.2011.01337.x

[7] Lu L, Hu Z, Frankel W, Shen R, Chen W, Pan X, et al. Using endoscopic optical coherence tomography to detect and treat early-stage pancreatic cancers. Frontiers in Oncology. 2021;**11**:591484. DOI: 10.3389/fonc.2021.591484

[8] Wang C, Qi X, Zhou X, Liu H, Li M. Diagnostic value of objective VELscope fluorescence methods in distinguishing oral cancer from oral potentially malignant disorders (OPMDs). Translational Cancer Research. 2022;**11**(6):1603. DOI: 10.21037/tcr-21-2804

[9] Huang D, Swanson EA, Lin CP, Schuman JS, Stinson WG, Chang W, et al. Optical coherence tomography. Science. 1991;**254**(5035):1178-1181. DOI: 10.1126/science.1957169

[10] Wilder-Smith P, Lee K, Guo S, Zhang J, Osann K, Chen Z, et al. In vivo diagnosis of oral dysplasia and malignancy using optical coherence tomography: Preliminary studies in 50 patients. Lasers in Surgery and Medicine: The Official Journal of the American Society for Laser Medicine and Surgery. 2009;**41**(5):353-357. DOI: 10.1002/lsm.20773

[11] Lee CK, Chi TT, Wu CT, Tsai MT, Chiang CP, Yang CC. Diagnosis of oral precancer with optical coherence tomography. Biomedical Optics Express. 2012;**3**(7):1632-1646. DOI: 10.1364/BOE.3.001632

[12] Jing J, Zhang J, Loy AC, Wong BJ, Chen Z. High-speed upper-airway imaging using full-range optical coherence tomography. Journal of Biomedical Optics. 2012;**17**(11):110507. DOI: 10.1117/1.JBO.17.11.110507

[13] Wang J, Xu Y, Boppart SA. Review of optical coherence tomography in

oncology. Journal of Biomedical Optics. 2017;**22**(12):121711. DOI: 10.1117/1.JBO.22.12.121711

[14] Chen XY, Zhou G, Zhang J. Optical coherence tomography: Promising imaging technique for the diagnosis of oral mucosal diseases. Oral Diseases. 2024;**30**(6):3638-3651. DOI: 10.1111/odi.14851

[15] Jing JC, Goshtasbi K, Wang Y, Chen JJ, Su E, Hong EM, et al. Optical coherence tomography to identify upper airway obstruction sites in an apneic patient. Biophotonics Discovery. 2024;**1**(3):035002. DOI: doi.org/10.1117/1.BIOS.1.3.035002

[16] Zhao Y, Chen Z, Saxer C, Xiang S, de Boer JF, Nelson JS. Phase-resolved optical coherence tomography and optical Doppler tomography for imaging blood flow in human skin with fast scanning speed and high velocity sensitivity. Optics Letters. 2000;**25**(2):114-116. DOI: 10.1364/OL.25.000114

[17] Bizheva K, Hosseinaee Z, Carter K, Hileeto D, Ballios BG, Sorbara L, et al. In vivo contactless, cellular-resolution imaging of the healthy and pathological human limbus with 250-kHz point-scanning SD-OCT. Translational Vision of science and Technology. 2024;**13**(12):29. DOI: 10.1167/tvst.13.12.29

[18] Sharma GK, Wong BJ. Optical coherence tomography of the oral cavity and pharynx: Normative anatomy and benign processes. In: Biomedical Optics in Otorhinolaryngology: Head and Neck Surgery. New York, NY: Springer New York; 2016. pp. 559-571. DOI: 10.1007/978-1-4939-1758-7_34

[19] Walther J, Golde J, Kirsten L. In vivo imaging of human oral hard and soft tissues by polarization-sensitive optical coherence tomography. Journal of Biomedical Optics. 2017;**22**(12):121717-121717. DOI: 10.1117/1.JBO.22.12.121717

[20] Leitgeb RA, Werkmeister RM, Blatter C. Doppler optical coherence tomography. Progress in Retinal and Eye Research. 2014;**41**:26-43. DOI: 10.1016/j.preteyeres.2014.03.004

[21] Choi WJ, Wang RK. In vivo imaging of functional microvasculature within tissue beds of oral and nasal cavities by swept-source optical coherence tomography with a forward/side-viewing probe. Biomedical Optics Express. 2014;**5**(8):2620-2634. DOI: 10.1364/BOE.5.002620

[22] Jing JC, Chou L, Su E. Anatomically correct visualization of the human upper airway using a high-speed long range optical coherence tomography system with an integrated positioning sensor. Scientific Reports. 2016;**6**(1):39443. DOI: 10.1038/srep39443

[23] Miao Y, Jing J, Chen Z. Graph-based rotational nonuniformity correction for localized compliance measurement in the human nasopharynx. Biomedical Optics Express. 2021;**12**(4):2508-2518. DOI: 10.1364/BOE.419997

[24] He Y, Shui H, Liu J. Neck dissection improves the prognosis of patients with early-stage oral squamous cell carcinoma. Scientific Reports. 2025;**15**(1):11640. DOI: 10.1038/s41598-025-96018-2

[25] Albano D, Argo A, Bilello G. Oral squamous cell carcinoma: Features and medico-legal implications of diagnostic omission. Case Reports in Dentistry. 2024;**2024**(1):2578271. DOI: 10.1155/2024/2578271

[26] Freilich MM, Epstein JB. The rising prevalence of oral potentially malignant disorders. Oral Health [Internet]. Toronto (ON): Oral Health Group; 13

Jan 2025. Available from: https://www.oralhealthgroup.com/features/the-rising-prevalence-of-oral-potentially-malignant-disorders/

[27] Gambino A, Martina E, Panzarella V, Ruggiero T, Haddad GE, Broccoletti R, et al. Potential use of optical coherence tomography in oral potentially malignant disorders: in-vivo case series study. BMC Oral Health. 2023;**23**(1):540. DOI: 10.1186/s12903-023-03263-w

[28] Panzarella V, Buttacavoli F, Gambino A, Capocasale G, Di Fede O, Mauceri R, et al. Site-coded oral squamous cell carcinoma evaluation by optical coherence tomography (OCT): A descriptive pilot study. Cancers. 2022;**14**(23):5916. DOI: 10.3390/cancers14235916

[29] Sunny SP, Agarwal S, James BL, Heidari E, Muralidharan A, Yadav V, et al. Intra-operative point-of-procedure delineation of oral cancer margins using optical coherence tomography. Oral Oncology. 2019;**92**:12-19. DOI: 10.1016/j.oraloncology.2019.03.006

[30] Yang Z, Shang J, Liu C, Zhang J, Liang Y. Identification of oral cancer in OCT images based on an optical attenuation model. Lasers in Medical Science. 2020;**35**:1999-2007. DOI: 10.1007/s10103-020-03025-y

[31] Jerjes W, Hamdoon Z, Rashed D, Hopper C. Advancing non-invasive diagnosis of oral epithelial dysplasia: Comparative insights from in vivo optical coherence tomography and histopathology. Journal of Clinical Medicine. 2025;**14**(4):1118. DOI: 10.3390/jcm14041118

[32] Jerjes W, Stevenson H, Ramsay D, Hamdoon Z. Enhancing Oral cancer detection: A systematic review of the diagnostic accuracy and future integration of optical coherence tomography with artificial intelligence. Journal of Clinical Medicine. 2024;**13**(19):5822. DOI: 10.3390/jcm13195822

[33] Heidari AE, Sunny SP, James BL, Lam TM, Tran AV, Yu J, et al. Optical coherence tomography as an oral cancer screening adjunct in a low resource settings. IEEE Journal of Selected Topics in Quantum Electronics. 2018;**25**(1):1-8. DOI: 10.1109/JSTQE.2018.2869643

[34] Das N, Sergey A, Zhou Y, Gilligan KE, Dwyer RM, Leahy M. Nanoscale structure detection and monitoring of tumour growth with optical coherence tomography. Nanoscale Advances. 2020;**2**(7):2853-2858. DOI: 10.1039/D0NA00371A

[35] Li JH, Du Y. The diagnosis of nasopharyngeal carcinoma by optical coherence tomography (OCT). Laser Physics. 2016;**26**(6):065003. DOI: 10.1088/1054-660X/26/6/065003

[36] Sun XM, Luo JQ, Xiao ZW, Gu QY, Lan LC, Zhang HQ, et al. Investigations on the potential of optical coherence tomography as an imaging tool for eustachian tube. Scientific Reports. 2021;**11**(1):8072. DOI: 10.1038/s41598-021-87637-6

[37] Young K, Ma E, Kejriwal S, Nielsen T, Aulakh SS, Birkeland AC. Intraoperative in vivo imaging modalities in head and neck cancer surgical margin delineation: A systematic review. Cancers. 2022;**14**(14):3416. DOI: 10.3390/cancers14143416

[38] Lee E, Chou L, Chen Z, Wong BJ. Optical imaging of cilia in the head and neck. Journal of Clinical Medicine. 2025;**14**(6):2059. DOI: 10.3390/jcm14062059

[39] Pan DW, Morán MA, Kim W, Yang Z, Applegate BE, Oghalai JS. Optical coherence tomography imaging and angiography of skull base tumors presenting as a middle ear mass in clinic. Diagnostics. 2025;**15**(6):732. DOI: 10.3390/diagnostics15060732

[40] Hill C, Malone J, Liu K, Ng SP, MacAulay C, Poh C, et al. Three-dimension epithelial segmentation in optical coherence tomography of the oral cavity using deep learning. Cancers. 2024;**16**(11):2144. DOI: 10.3390/cancers16112144

[41] Yuan W, Rao J, Liu Y, Li S, Qin L, Huang X. Deep radiomics-based prognostic prediction of oral cancer using optical coherence tomography. BMC Oral Health. 2024;**24**(1):1117. DOI: 10.1186/s12903-024-04849-8

[42] Malone J, Hill C, Tanskanen A, Liu K, Ng S, MacAulay C, et al. Imaging biomarkers of oral dysplasia and carcinoma measured with in vivo endoscopic optical coherence tomography. Cancers. 2024;**16**(15):2751. DOI: 10.3390/cancers16152751

[43] Chan KA, Woo JK, King A, Zee BC, Lam WJ, Chan SL, et al. Analysis of plasma Epstein–Barr virus DNA to screen for nasopharyngeal cancer. New England Journal of Medicine. 2017;**377**(6):513-522. DOI: 10.1056/NEJMoa1701717

[44] Chen WJ, Yu X, Lu YQ, Pfeiffer RM, Ling W, Xie SH, et al. Impact of an Epstein-Barr virus serology-based screening program on nasopharyngeal carcinoma mortality: A cluster-randomized controlled trial. Journal of Clinical Oncology. 2025;**43**(1):22-31. DOI: 10.1200/JCO.23.01296

Chapter 2

Role of Circulating Tumor DNA (ctDNA) in Head and Neck Squamous Cell Carcinoma

Mallory McKeon, Megha Mohanakrishnan, Priscilla F.A. Pichardo, Alice L. Tang, Chad A. Zender and Dustin A. Silverman

Abstract

Head and neck cancer is the sixth most common cancer worldwide with classically poor outcomes related to advanced disease at presentation. Despite improvements in treatment strategies, morbidity and mortality remain high among this patient population, with frequent disease recurrence and need for lifelong surveillance. Oropharyngeal squamous cell carcinoma (OPSCC), a disease historically associated with alcohol and tobacco abuse, has become increasingly prevalent in young, otherwise healthy patients related to chronic infection with human papillomavirus (HPV). Though this subset of patients has favorable response to therapy, patients' young age and health status places them at higher risk for delayed diagnosis and represents a challenge for long-term cancer surveillance. Circulating tumor DNA (ctDNA) has recently gained traction as a potential surveillance tool and affords the opportunity to shift this paradigm. Herein, we delve into the current, though constantly evolving, knowledge surrounding ctDNA and its role in the management of patients with HPV-mediated squamous cell carcinoma of the head and neck.

Keywords: circulating tumor DNA (ctDNA), human papillomavirus (HPV), oropharyngeal squamous cell carcinoma, biomarkers, liquid biopsy

1. Introduction

Head and neck cancer represents a highly challenging disease with profound impacts on patients and families [1, 2]. Rates of diagnosis remain high and accounted for approximately 950,000 cases of all diagnosed cancers and 468,000 cancer deaths globally in 2022, representing about 5% of all cancers worldwide [3]. While many treatment advances have been realized over the past several decades, survival rates among this cohort have remained steady, and further underscores the challenges associated with successful management [4]. Although the traditional risk factors such as tobacco and alcohol abuse have been attributed to the majority of head and neck cancers within the United States, human papillomavirus (HPV) has been identified as the causative oncogenic factor in the development of oropharyngeal squamous cell carcinoma (OPSCC) with a distinct diagnosis, treatment, and surveillance profile compared to other subsites within the head and neck [5–8].

OPSCC is defined as the subset of cancers that encompasses the palatine tonsils, base of tongue, soft palate, and uvula. HPV is a rising independent risk factor associated with OPSCC, once accounting for 15% of cases in the 1980s compared to more than 70% during the 2000s; alarmingly, this number continues to rise [5, 9]. Due to its rising incidence, the American Joint Committee on Cancer (AJCC) highlighted the importance of distinguishing HPV-positive from HPV-negative OPSCC due to differences in unique molecular profiles and treatment outcomes [10]. Overall, this subset of head and neck cancer responds better to both uni- and multimodal treatment with improved prognosis compared to non-HPV-mediated tumors [11]. Moreover, studies have demonstrated that patients with HPV-mediated OPSCC have favorable disease outcomes despite being often diagnosed at advanced clinical stages [12]. As such, current management paradigms are increasingly designed to identify patients at earlier stages of disease and select those at risk for recurrence and distant metastases. To accomplish this, increased attention to biomarkers, specifically circulating tumor DNA (ctDNA), has emerged as a central target in the effort to improve diagnostic and treatment outcomes for this population.

2. HPV pathogenesis

HPV is a non-enveloped virus with circular double-stranded DNA that replicates in stratified epithelial layers. It often infects the basal layer of the epithelium, exposed by a cutaneous skin injury, and its viral lifecycle works concurrently with the migration of the epithelial cells toward the surface. HPV lacks its own enzymes for DNA replication and instead relies on those of its epithelial cell host [13].

The most common mutation associated with head and neck cancer involves the TP53 gene [14]. TP53 is an important tumor suppressor gene that helps to regulate cellular replication. Specifically, p53—a tumor suppressor protein produced by TP53—responds to cell stress or DNA injury by initiating growth arrest, DNA repair, or apoptosis [15]. Consequently, aberrations in TP53 perpetuate high rates of growth and dedifferentiation in cancer cells. Though a TP53 mutation is seen in up to 81% of HPV-negative oropharyngeal cancer samples, one study found that TP53 mutations were only seen in about 4% of HPV-positive squamous cell carcinoma cases [16]. Though these values vary across studies, it is accepted that HPV-mediated cancers generally have fewer mutations than cancers caused by tobacco and alcohol. This may be attributable to viral E proteins, which directly target cell defense mechanisms [17]. For example, E6 directly inhibits p53 by binding to a ubiquitin-protein ligase and promoting its breakdown [18]. Thus, viral proteins effectively disrupt cell cycle regulation without relying on somatic mutations. In addition, HPV-positive tumors demonstrate mutations that impede a cell's ability to repair damage, regulate transcription, and signal to the body that the cell has been compromised [19]. Specific to HPV-mediated oropharyngeal cancer, PIK3Ca and KMT2D oncogenic mutations are more common, followed by CASP8, FBXW7 and FBXW8 (**Table 1**) [14].

At the basal layer, the viral oncoproteins E6 and E7, in conjunction, promote epithelial cell proliferation and differentiation. E7 binds with the retinoblastoma

Mutation	Mechanism of Carcinogenesis/Clinical Significance	% observed in HPV+ OPSCC
TP53	Tumor suppressor gene triggers DNA repair or autophagy in response to cell damage. Most common mutation in non-HPV-mediated OPSCC (up to 85%)	4–31% [7, 12]
PIK3CA	Important for cell growth and division; proto-oncogene when mutated, leading to uncontrolled replication	17–31% [7, 12, 20]
KMT2D	Tumor suppressor, important for histone methylation	10–24% [7, 12]
NOTCH1	Important for cell differentiation; more commonly mutated (16%) in HPV-negative disease	7.4%
TERT	Telomerase reverse transcriptase; inappropriately lengthens telomeres when mutated, influencing cell lifetime, proliferation, and gene expression. More commonly mutated (32%) in HPV-negative disease	0%
HPV DNA	Uses E proteins (primarily E6 and E7) to promote cell growth and dysregulate replication	100%

Abbreviations: Human papillomavirus (HPV), oropharyngeal squamous cell carcinoma (OPSCC).

Table 1.
Oncogenic mutations in oropharyngeal squamous cell carcinoma.

tumor suppressor gene (pRB) which typically regulates the G1/S progression in the cell cycle. Normally, at G1, pRB is bound to E2F, a transcription factor activator, and represses its activity. Cyclin-dependent kinases eventually join and phosphorylate pRB, removing its binding to E2F and allowing for the transition to the S-phase, where DNA transcription occurs. However, the E7 protein may preferentially bind to pRB and disassociate the pRB/E2F complex earlier, thus promoting HPV transcription and dysregulating the epithelial cell cycle. In high-risk HPV subtypes, it is also found that the oncogenic interaction of E7 and pRB promotes the stabilization of p53 (a tumor suppressor protein) and causes cell apoptosis. Therefore, E6 plays a role in p53 degradation, preventing cell death in those expressing E7 [13, 21–23]. In the middle epithelial layers, viral genome amplification proteins, such as E4, are activated. Finally, in the upper epithelial layers, the structural capsid proteins L1 and L2 are triggered by the HPV-infected cells to assist in viral packaging and the eventual release of the virus [13].

Importantly, a tumor is classified as HPV-positive if it expresses HPV E6/E7 mRNA or if HPV DNA is detected along with its surrogate biomarker, p16. In HPV-mediated OPSCC, the overactivation of E6 and E7 proteins drives carcinogenesis. Similarly, the suppression of E2, a viral transcription repressor that regulates E6 and E7 activity, is also observed in those with HPV-positive OPSCC [23]. Importantly, in HPV-mediated tumor cells, p53 function may still be functionally intact despite its dysregulation by viral oncoproteins [24]. From a treatment perspective, radiation therapy has been demonstrated to reinstate the apoptotic pathways in these cancers and lead to therapeutic effects [25]. Similarly, a study focused on chemotherapy outcomes on HPV-mediated tumors using cisplatin resulted in strong repression of viral E6 and E7 oncogene expression and eventually resulted in apoptotic cell death of HPV-positive cancer cells (**Figure 1**). While these pathways remain critical to the current understanding of OPSCC pathogenesis, the reliability of detecting these mutations is eclipsed by that of ctHPV DNA in the context of virally-mediated cancer, which is present and detectable in 99–100% of samples from patients with HPV-mediated oropharyngeal cancer [26].

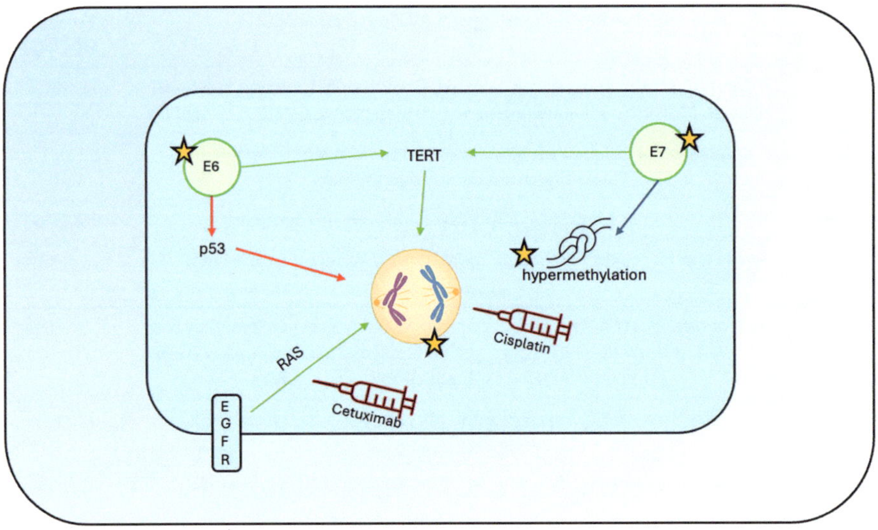

Figure 1.
Mechanisms of carcinogenesis in HPV-mediated oropharyngeal squamous cell carcinoma. Carcinogenesis is primarily driven by E6 and E7 viral proteins, though there are several viral proteins that contribute to cellular stability and abnormal growth patterns. In the diagram, the green arrow represents amplification while the red arrow represents inhibition. Here, the relationship between viral proteins and chemotherapeutic agents is highlighted.

3. Current landscape of HPV-mediated OPSCC

Compared to tobacco and alcohol abuse as the common risk factors for the development of head and neck cancer more broadly, unique risk factors for the development of HPV-mediated OPSCCs include multiple sexual partners and practices that involve oral sexual intercourse, as these increase the likelihood of HPV exposure [27]. While HPV-positive OPSCC is more prevalent among those abstaining from tobacco and alcohol consumption, patients with a significant use history experience worse outcomes compared to their tobacco and alcohol-free counterparts [28].

Specifically, over 80% of all HPV-positive OPSCCs arise from HPV-16, a high-risk subtype of HPV for which prophylactic vaccines are available [5]. Other well-studied causative high-risk HPV subtypes include HPV 18, 31, 33, and 35 [29]. A landmark retrospective analysis by Ang et al. demonstrated that tumor HPV status was a strong and independent prognostic factor for patients with OPSCC with 3-year overall survival rates of 82.4 versus 57.1% among those with HPV-positive and HPV-negative tumors, respectively. Further, HPV tumor positivity was found to be associated with a 58% reduction in the risk of death compared to HPV-negative disease following adjustment for age, race, tumor and nodal stage, tobacco exposure, and treatment type [30].

Current treatments for HPV-mediated OPSCC include surgery, radiation therapy (RT), chemotherapy, immunotherapy, and a combination of these modalities. Previously, due to the difficulty in accessing sites of primary OPSCC, surgical resection was traditionally accomplished through larger and more invasive transoral, transpharyngeal, or transmandibular approaches. The morbidity associated with such approaches has the potential to result in increased rates of postoperative speech, swallowing, and breathing deficits. The introduction of minimally invasive alternatives such as transoral laser microsurgery (TLM) and transoral robotics surgery (TORS) has revolutionized treatment paradigms for this population and resulted in improved functional outcomes while maintaining oncologic success, particularly among those with early-stage disease [31].

While recent efforts have focused on treatment de-escalation strategies among those with HPV-mediated disease, significant controversy regarding appropriate patient selection and optimal therapeutic approaches exists [32]. The identification of new prognostic factors, particularly the incorporation of molecular biomarkers such as ctDNA is central to defining these parameters and potentially identifying patients that may benefit from treatment de-escalation or escalation. Importantly, ctDNA has shown recent promise as a tool for improvement in head and neck cancer diagnosis, treatment response, and surveillance [33]. As such, a deeper understanding of the role of ctDNA in head and neck cancer treatment is warranted.

4. ctDNA detection methods

Unique to head and neck cancers, ctDNA can be obtained through saliva sampling, oral wash, plasma, and serum—so-called "liquid biopsies." Not surprisingly, oral washing has the highest sensitivity among oral cavity cancers (100% sensitivity versus 47–70% for other head and neck subsites) [34]. In oropharyngeal cancer, plasma samples were much more likely (91%) to detect ctDNA than saliva (47%) (**Figure 2**) [35]. Combining multiple sampling methods improved results across multiple studies [34–37].

Two predominant detection methods for identifying ctDNA exist: isolated polymerase chain reaction (PCR)-based techniques and BEAMing (beads, emulsion, amplification, and magnetic), which combines PCR and flow cytometry. Pure PCR detection may utilize digital PCR (dPCR) or droplet digital PCR (ddPCR). In the setting of OPSCC, ddPCR is generally preferred for its higher sensitivity, achieved *via* an emulsification process that eliminates the need for serial dilution, which can contribute to false negative results [36]. PCR overall is highly sensitive and is reliable for detecting known oncogenes, including E6 and E7 proteins. BEAMing utilizes magnetic beads after amplification to divide DNA molecules prior to flow cytometry. This three

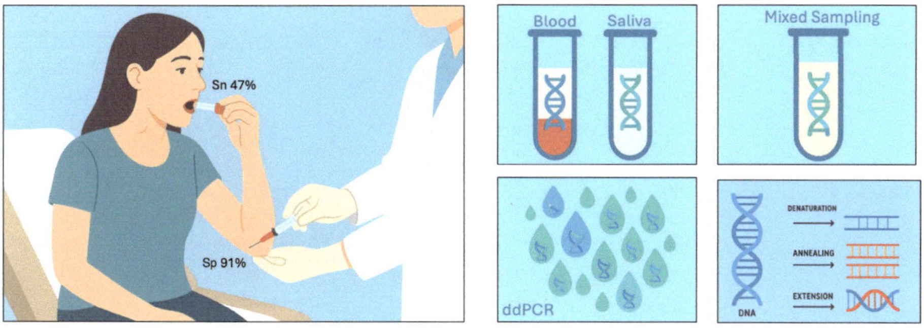

Figure 2.
ctDNA as a Liquid Biopsy Technique. ctDNA may be detected in saliva or in blood samples. In the setting of oropharyngeal cancer, the sensitivity is higher for blood sampling (91 vs. 47%), though both are characterized by high (91%) specificity. Mixed sampling is recommended to increase the test's sensitivity. After samples are obtained, amplification is completed. Abbreviations: Sensitivity (Sn), Specificity (Sp), droplet digital polymerase chain reaction (ddPCR).

step process enables BEAMing to detect alleles as rare as 0.0001% allele frequency [36]. Both PCR and BEAMing are limited in that they require targeted genes for testing. Next-generation sequencing (NGS) and methylation profiling present unique opportunities to examine ctDNA more broadly. Methylation studies demonstrated lower sensitivity and specificity than targeted detection methods [38]. Conversely, in direct comparison to quantitative PCR and ddPCR, NGS has the highest overall sensitivity and specificity for detecting HPV-mediated cancers [39]. However, NGS is not without its limitations; typically, it can only sequence DNA segments of approximately 200 base pairs [40]. Whole genome sequencing is less cost-effective and may present new challenges with mutations of unknown clinical significance.

Viral-DNA overcomes the limitations of PCR and BEAMing by providing a dependable target for diagnostic testing. There are several available tests specific to HPV-mediated ctDNA on the market (**Table 2**). Signatera™ (Natera) is a panel of somatic variants based on the most common mutation profiles encountered in HPV-mediated OPSCC. This was demonstrated to be highly reliable in detecting minimal residual disease in patients with detectable mutations at the time of diagnosis, which included 75% of patients in its primary study [41]. Alternatively, NavDx® (Naveris) and Guardant360® measure viral HPV DNA in patients' plasma. NavDx® has the most robust data, with pre-treatment sensitivity ranging 91 to 98% and surveillance sensitivity of 81–88%; specificity is 100% in either setting [42, 43]. NavDx® tests for the five most common cancer causing strains of HPV (16, 18, 31, 33, and 35—responsible for approximately 90% of HPV-mediated oropharyngeal cancer), making it a strong initial test for patients with suspected HPV-mediated oropharyngeal cancer [42–44]. In contrast, Guardant360®, which tests for a broader array of oncogenic

Test	What it measures	Clinical relevance (HPV+ OPSCC)	Reported performance	Price
NavDx® (Naveris)	ctHPV DNA (16/18/31/33/35) in plasma	Pre-treatment detection, Surveillance, MRD	Pre-treatment: Sn ~91–98%, Sp 100% Surveillance: Sn ~82–88%, Sp 100% PPV ~100%;	ADLT $1800; Medicare covered for OPSCC surveillance; OOP: $50–$150
Guardant360® (Liquid)	Tumor NGS HPV/ EBV DNA (14 HPV strains)	Genomic profiling in advanced disease; not validated for OPC surveillance	Sn 93.6%, Sp 96.6%	ADLT and listed OOP $5000; $3000–$3100; OOP assistance available
Signatera™ (Natera)	Somatic ctDNA (patient-specific variants), not HPV DNA	MRD/recurrence tracking when mutation-based assay is preferred	Detected 75% known disease (pre-treatment) Detected MRD, predicted recurrence	ADLT $3920; Medicare coverage; ~$100 s OOP with assistance programs

Abbreviations: Human papillomavirus (HPV), Sensitivity (Sn), specificity (Sp), Advanced Diagnostic Laboratory Test (ADLT); Out-of-Pocket Payers (OOP), Minimum residual disease (MRD), Next-generation sequencing (NGS), oropharyngeal squamous cell carcinoma (OPSCC).

Table 2.
Comparison of ctDNA Assays.

virus strains including Epstein-Barr virus (EBV), but has not yet been validated in HPV-mediated OPSCC. It also has reduced sensitivity in indolent tumors, making it a less reliable test for early detection or surveillance [45].

5. ctDNA utility in oropharyngeal squamous cell carcinoma

5.1 ctDNA at diagnosis

As previously outlined, there are inherent limitations to detecting somatic mutations in ctDNA for detecting and monitoring cancer [26]. By directly testing for HPV DNA, specificity and sensitivity are both increased—up to 98% for both [46]. One highly reliable and best first test for patients presenting with a concern for oropharyngeal malignancy is fine needle aspiration (FNA) biopsy, particularly for those presenting with a neck mass of unclear etiology, which has a sensitivity of approximately 74% [47]. Recently, Chernesky et al. explored the utility of testing FNA samples for HPV E6, rather than the conventional p16 staining [48]. In 59 patients with HPV-mediated OPSCC, 81% tested positive *via* immunohistochemistry and 80% were positive for HPV E6/E7 mRNA and DNA, showing comparable results. In this study, both tests required adequate tissue sampling for diagnosis, which may represent a challenge for patients presenting with a necrotic metastatic lymph node. In low-resource settings, tissue samples may also be compromised by access to the appropriate needles, slides, preservation techniques, and storage capabilities, making histologic diagnosis more difficult [40]. Similarly, a 2021 meta-analysis compared the accuracy of tissue biopsy to blood (e.g. liquid biopsy) and salivary samples, finding the former two comparable (sensitivity ~81% and specificity ~95%) [49].

Obtaining plasma ctDNA is a less invasive method of accurate cancer biomarker detection and represents an opportunity in expediting appropriate oncologic care. Several series have demonstrated that 90% of patients had detectable ctDNA at the time of diagnosis with new HPV-mediated OPSCC [46]. One study retrospectively detected HPV ctDNA in blood samples obtained several years before patients' cancer was clinically detectable [36, 50]. Though the practical application of this approach warrants careful consideration, the data clearly support that liquid biopsies have potential value in diagnosing and monitoring HPV-mediated head and neck cancer, a disease process that has otherwise been challenging to detect at early onset. Further, if levels of ctDNA may be consistently correlated to disease stage, similar tests may be incorporated as a useful adjunct in counseling patients and families on treatment plans (**Figure 3**).

Unlike FNA or primary tumor biopsies, liquid biopsy *via* ctHPVDNA provides valuable quantitative data correlating to disease burden. Cao et al. showed prognostic value in both pre-treatment baselines and peri-treatment levels [51]. The literature consistently supports that ctDNA levels at the time of diagnosis correlate with tumor size and burden [34, 38, 52, 53]. One prospective study of 72 patients with HPV-mediated OPSCC highlighted a direct correlation between baseline HPV DNA levels and AJCC cancer stage [20]. Subsequent studies have similarly shown a strong correlation between quantitative ctHPV DNA and tumor size or stage [38, 46, 54, 55]. As such, the sensitivity of ctDNA increases in advanced disease [38]. Several authors have also suggested that levels may be indicative of lymph node burden and could have potential application for detecting distant metastasis in the absence of locoregional recurrence [38, 56, 57]. Yin et al. discovered early postoperative detection of ctDNA may be associated with nodal disease burden, including size of largest node

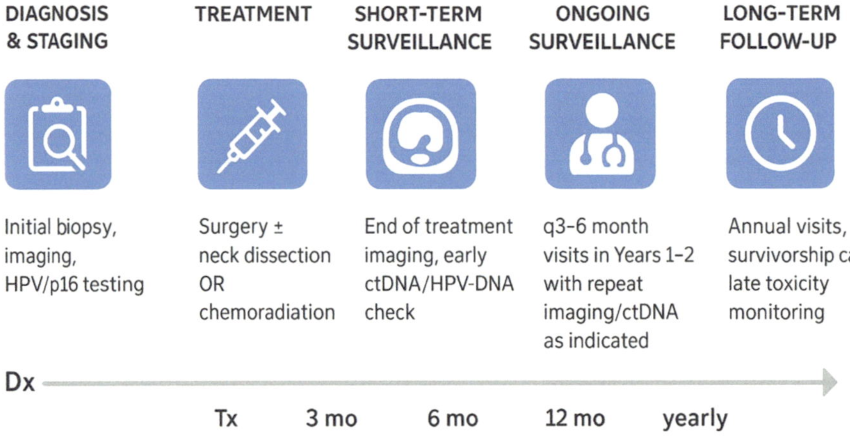

Figure 3.
The role of ctDNA throughout each phase of oncologic care.

and number of lymph nodes involved [57]. These findings have potential downstream implications for patient counseling, raising the question of whether quantified ctDNA should be considered in surgical planning and treatment selection.

5.2 Assessing treatment response

A salient benefit of liquid biopsies is their ability to provide real-time data on tumor burden; though ctDNA kinetics vary across tumor subtypes, there is reliable clearance following definitive surgery [58]. Postoperative testing can identify minimal residual disease (MRD) [58]. Classically, post-treatment positron emission tomography (PET) is utilized to assess for MRD and identify patients that require further testing and treatment. To mitigate the confounding effect of inflammation on PET imaging, scans are typically obtained at 12 weeks following completion of primary treatment. At present, we do not know the half-life of ctDNA in HPV-mediated OPSCC. In other cancer types such as colorectal, lung, and nasopharyngeal carcinoma, the half-life of ctDNA ranges 0.5–2.0 hours [58]. Preliminary studies have found that ctDNA from HPV-related oropharynx cancer is cleared within 3 days of surgery [58]. Huttinger et al. echoed these findings and demonstrated that clearance of ctDNA following induction chemotherapy more accurately predicted response to therapy than PET imaging in a cohort of 17 patients [56]. These results were confirmed by Berger et al. [59] In the largest study to date, authors showed that 98% of patients with detectable ctDNA following definitive treatment had evidence of residual or recurrent disease at the first follow-up encounter. Thus, ctDNA could feasibly be applied months earlier than PET imaging to determine MRD or recurrence after treatment. Notably, these findings and incorporation of ctDNA into future management and surveillance protocols may meaningfully guide earlier interventions and clinical decision-making regarding receipt of adjuvant treatments.

Similarly, clearance of ctHPV DNA after definitive chemoradiation (CRT) therapy was a better indicator of response to treatment and predictor of recurrence than post-treatment PET imaging [44]. The kinetics of ctDNA are more complicated during primary CRT than following surgery given the mechanisms and chronicity of treatment. One study found that an initial rise in ctDNA is favorable for overall treatment response and may represent a cellular senescence phase [51]. Another associated favorable long-term outcomes in patients who had cleared greater than 95% of their baseline ctDNA by day 28 of treatment [51, 52]. Though larger series are warranted to further elucidate ctDNA trends during and following CRT, these results are promising for an early, or peri-treatment mechanism for monitoring treatment response and may guide treatment escalation or de-escalation in some circumstances. As such,

Author	No.	Test	Sensitivity	Specificity	Primary Conclusions	Limitations
Ahn et al. 2014 [37]	93	ddPCR E6/E7	69%	90%	Combines plasma and saliva testing to improve surveillance; associated post-treatment level with survival	Retrospective
Chera et al. 2019 [52]	103	ddPCR HPV DNA	89%	97%	Correlates rapid clearance with disease control and prognosis	Limited long-term data included
Hanna et al. 2019 [60]	21	ddPCR for HPV DNA in plasma and saliva	87%	67%	Salivary HPV DNA correlates with disease burden in OPC	Small sample size, observational
Rettig et al. 2022 [61]	196	TTMV-HPV DNA	69%	96%	Post-treatment positivity associated with reduced survival	Small samples of N0 cancer and surgical patients
Siravegna et al. 2022 [26]	70	ddPCR	98%	98%	ctDNA is a reliable, cost-effective, and rapid tool	Observational design, single institution, moderate sample
Ferrandino et al. 2023 [42]	399	TTMV-HPV DNA assay	88%	100%	Demonstrated utility of HPV DNA testing in diagnosis and surveillance	Retrospective cohort study, missing baseline levels
Campo et al. 2024 [62]	1311	ddPCR	86%	96%	Liquid biopsy has potential for earlier diagnosis of primary and recurrent cancer	Heterogeneity in testing/timing
Kais et al. 2024 [63]	27	ddPCR	96%	100%	ctDNA has potential to expedite diagnosis and treatment of occult primary	Small sample size, single institution

Abbreviations: droplet digital polymerase chain reaction (ddPCR), tumor tissue modified viral HPV DNA (TTMV-HPV-DNA), circulating tumor DNA (ctDNA).

Table 3.
Utility of Circulating Tumor DNA (ctDNA) in Selected Series.

several studies are ongoing to investigate the role of ctDNA in de-escalation of treatment [40]. **Table 3** tabulates the utility of ctDNA testing across selected series.

Mutation profiling through ctDNA may also guide treatment paradigms. For example, prospective de-escalation trials are actively exploring the role of liquid biopsy in treatment counseling. Chen et al. studied patients with HPV-related OPSCC following surgical resection who had biochemical clearance of tumor tissue modified viral (TTMV) HPV DNA (measured *via* NavDx®) [64]. In this study, complete resection was determined by postoperative magnetic resonance imaging (MRI). Patients with one pathologic risk factor warranting adjuvant therapy and the absence of gross residual disease by postoperative MRI and TTMV-HPV DNA were closely monitored. Unfortunately, three patients developed biochemical or radiographic evidence of recurrence warranting delayed adjuvant radiotherapy, and the study was prematurely closed.

Mutation profiling with ctDNA may also provide crucial information regarding susceptibility or resistance to targeted chemotherapy. For instance, cetuximab (a monoclonal antibody that targets epidermal growth factor receptor [EGFR]) is commonly utilized in combination with platinum-based agents for the treatment of locoregionally advanced head and neck cancer. Unfortunately, patients with head and neck cancer may develop resistance to cetuximab. In the setting of colorectal cancer, acquired resistance to cetuximab is understood to occur through mutations involving EGFR or downstream regulators in the RAS pathway [65, 66]. Braig et al. investigated 46 patients with head and neck cancer (11% with HPV-mediated OPSCC) treated with cetuximab; overall, one-third of their participants acquired RAS mutations during cetuximab therapy, which was detected using NGS of ctDNA in peripheral blood samples [65]. All RAS mutations were associated with disease progression, suggesting an association between constitutively activated RAS and cetuximab resistance [65].

5.3 ctDNA as a surveillance tool

Some series have raised concerns regarding the reliability of ctDNA in the detection of MRD. The limiting factor for liquid biopsy is the lowest detectable mutant allele fraction [38]. As noted in prior sections of this chapter, the sensitivity of ctDNA testing directly correlated to disease burden. From this, one may extrapolate that states of lower disease burden—including the early stages of recurrence—pose a diagnostic challenge. Despite these concerns, evidence supports the utility of ctDNA in cancer surveillance (**Figures 4** and **5**). Chera et al. (2020) examined 1006 blood samples across 115 patients with HPV-mediated OPSCC and demonstrated that those with undetectable ctDNA following treatment with curative intent had >99% negative predictive value for remission [46]. Conversely, 94% of patients with positive post-treatment ctDNA later recurred [46]. Though the kinetics of ctDNA remain ill-defined, Efthymiou et al. 2024 found that ctDNA was predictive of recurrence across all tumor types [58]. In a similar study, Jakobsen et al. identified recurrent HPV-mediated cancer in 8 of 13 patients with persistent ctDNA positivity after treatment [49]. Notably, the five patients in Jakobsen's study with positive ctDNA and no clinical evidence of recurrence after up to 25 months of follow-up highlight the need for improved understanding of ctDNA kinetics.

Yin et al. (2025) prospectively evaluated ctDNA kinetics in 57 patients with known pre-treatment positivity at two distinct time points (1–2 days postoperative and 2 weeks postoperative) [57]. Sixteen patients in their study had detectable HPV DNA at postoperative day 1–2; three quarters of those resolved by week two, leading the authors to recommend waiting to draw baseline postoperative labs until 2 weeks after

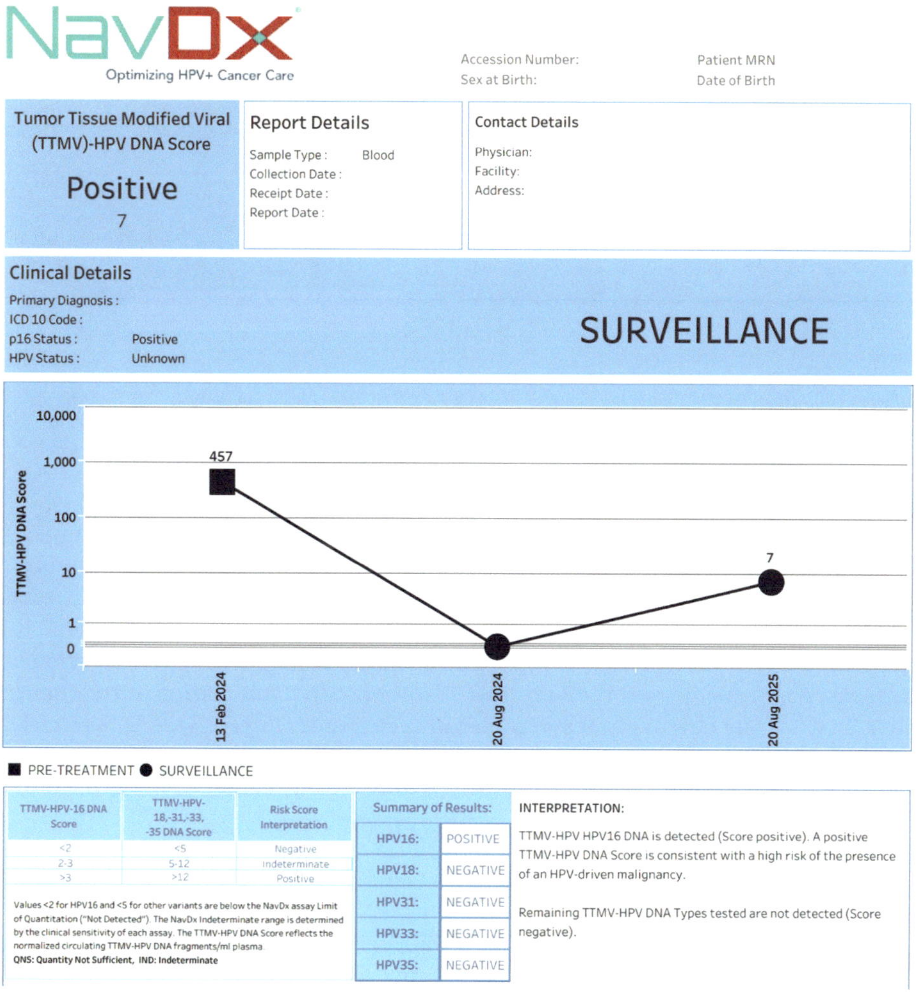

Figure 4.
NavDx® (Naveris) Surveillance TTMV-HPV Test. A patient with a history of cT3N1 HPV-mediated oropharyngeal squamous cell carcinoma underwent definitive chemoradiation treatment. Baseline pre-treatment NavDx TTMV-HPV DNA score was 457, which declined to undetectable levels 3 months following completion of therapy. Subsequent surveillance testing 1 year following definitive CRT demonstrated a detectable increase with TTMV-HPV DNA score of 7, consistent with biopsy-proven recurrence.

surgery. The four patients whose HPV DNA levels remained detectable at 2 weeks had persistent positive labs until the initiation of advent therapy, at which point all levels abated [57]. All patients in this study were followed for 24 months. The four patients who ultimately required adjuvant therapy remained disease-free during that period. Two patients developed recurrence—one of whom had detectable HPVDNA at postoperative day 1–2 and one who did not; both did demonstrate steadily rising levels of HPV DNA preceding clinical or radiographic recurrence [57].

The literature consistently supports that biochemical recurrence is evident before radiographic or clinical evidence [42, 50, 54]. In one study, a liquid biopsy detected evidence of recurrence 3.9 months before radiographic evidence [57]. Ferrandino et al. found that ctDNA demonstrated biochemical evidence of recurrence on average 47 days before pathologic confirmation and an earliest lead time of 520 days [42].

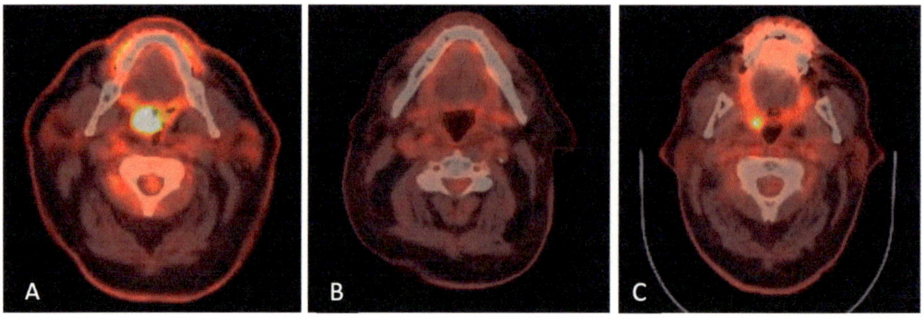

Figure 5.
PET-avid right oropharyngeal HPV-mediated squamous cell carcinoma. Patient from **Figure 4**. *(A) Pre-treatment axial fused PET/CT image demonstrating an avid (SUV 9.6) right oropharyngeal HPV-mediated cT3N1 tumor. (B) Three-month post-treatment PET imaging demonstrating marked interval resolution of previously demonstrated right oropharyngeal primary tumor (SUV 2.7). (C) 12-month surveillance PET/CT demonstrating a new FDG-avid right oropharyngeal HPV-mediated recurrence (SUV 6.7).*

However, the literature lacks a standardized approach to monitoring. For example, Yin et al. recommend baseline measurements at 2 weeks post-op, while Efthymiou et al. suggest 3 days [57, 58]. The National Cancer Institute Task Force for Colorectal Cancer presents a standardized algorithm measuring ctDNA in the setting of colorectal cancer—each timepoint with distinct goals of monitoring; these include: at diagnosis, post-neoadjuvant therapy, post-resection, after completion of treatment, and at onset of any new signs or symptoms of recurrence (**Figure 3**) [67]. Similarly, Campo et al. call for a standardized algorithm of surveillance testing, utilizing meta-analysis to depict how a multimodal approach to cancer surveillance could shift the landscape of head and neck surveillance more broadly.

5.4 Cancer of unknown primary (CUP)

One potential emerging application of ctDNA is in establishing HPV status in head and neck CUP. A new and enlarging neck mass is a common chief complaint with new patient presentations to head and neck cancer clinics and represents the most common presentation of HPV-mediated OPSCC. However, in the absence of a clearly defined primary tumor, patients have historically been empirically treated with broad-field radiation to ensure appropriate coverage and eradication of occult disease. In an important pilot study, Kais et al. showed that in 14 patients with CUP, FNA was non-diagnostic in two, and standard HPV testing with immunohistochemistry staining and in-situ hybridization failed to detect HPV in 7 of 12 and 4 of 7 patients, respectively [63]. In the same cohort, ctDNA had a 100% positive predictive value. If integrated into current diagnostic algorithms, ctDNA has the potential to reduce the number of procedures required and the time to treatment for patients with head and neck CUP, though further studies are warranted. Currently, neither the College of American Pathologists nor the American Society of Clinical Oncology encourages the use of ctDNA testing in clinical counseling for squamous cell carcinoma of unknown primary site [68, 69].

6. ctDNA cost

Reportedly, manufacturers had previously marketed gene testing, including ctDNA, direct-to-consumer at a cost of approximately $700 [70]. However, US

Federal Drug Administration has subsequently forbidden this, labeling the test as a type of medical device that cannot be safely and meaningfully interpreted without board-certified physicians [70]. The cost of ctDNA testing is presently set by Advanced Diagnostic Laboratory Test (ADLT) standards [54]. This refers to market pricing for lab-sourced testing of novel tests (e.g., data that cannot be obtained from standard hospital-run lab tests). Prices are initially set based on the manufacturer's listed price; after 9 months on the market, the price is reset annually to the median private-payer rate as reported by the lab. Cost to out-of-pocket (OOP) payers is typically much lower. ddPCR is an expensive test, particularly in low-resource settings.

Though NGS and ddPCR are typically high-cost, the targeted nature of HPV-specific diagnostics, such as NavDx®, makes them more cost-effective [54]. Current market prices based on ADLT are listed in **Table 3**. Kowalchuk et al. estimated the cost of ctDNA surveillance testing for HPV-mediated OPSCC to be approximately $500 [71]. In the same review, PET imaging and computed tomography scans of the head and neck are estimated to cost $7290 to $8710 and $2260 to $3030, respectively [71]. Not only is radiography expensive, but tests may also subject patients to radiation and potentially nephrotoxic contrast material, especially important considerations for those with end-stage renal disease or other contrast-related allergies. These risks would be mitigated by implementing non-invasive disease testing and monitoring through ctDNA. Siravegna et al. concluded that such an approach to diagnosis of HPV-mediated OPSCC using ctHPV DNA was 36–38% less expensive than today's standard clinical workup [70]. The additional cost benefits throughout lifelong surveillance were not included in this analysis; however, others have also emphasized the potential for liquid biopsies to dramatically lower economic barriers in surveillance of such cancers [71, 72].

There are inevitable indirect costs associated with cancer care that are unrelated to the actual price tag of medical care. Time lost from work, either due to fragility during treatment or related to direct clinical care (hospitalization, clinic visits, etc.), may generate a significant burden on patients' professional lives and result in further financial toxicity [73]. The integration of ctDNA to disease surveillance may conceivably reduce indirect costs of cancer surveillance by supplementing the need for imaging and serial examinations. Should the literature prove true, ctDNA may also detect cancer recurrence at earlier stages and further mitigate the morbidity and mortality of patients with recurrent and/or metastatic head and neck cancer. Finally, though having a reliable non-invasive method of monitoring cancer recurrence is unlikely to replace or eliminate the need for cross-sectional imaging or more invasive diagnostic procedures, it may mollify the emotional turmoil of living in remission by providing a checkpoint and adjunct test to utilize at the onset of rising patient concerns. Of course, this should be done thoughtfully and in the context of understanding testing limitations.

7. ctDNA limitations and future directions

Overall, the existing literature is constrained by several important methodological and clinical limitations. Most studies to date have involved small sample sizes, often pilot or observational in nature, with limited follow-up. Due to the population of focus, it is challenging to develop controlled studies, thereby restricting generalizability. Further, diagnostic performance has not been comprehensively evaluated, precluding validation of long-term outcomes. Considerable heterogeneity in study design, timing of assays, and performance characteristics underscores the imminent need for larger, prospective validation studies. Importantly, most studies do not adequately account for clinical features of the disease, and there remains no standardized pathway or algorithm for determining the optimal timing of liquid biopsies and HPV DNA sampling—whether in the immediate perioperative period, at 3 months, or at regular testing and surveillance intervals. Finally, while enthusiasm is growing for the incorporation of ctDNA testing into prospective clinical trials, robust integration into trial design and real-world clinical practice has not yet been achieved.

8. Conclusions

ctDNA has emerged as a clinically relevant tool with rapidly evolving applications in head and neck oncology, though its optimal role in guiding appropriate management is continues to evolve. ctDNA assays are increasingly applied across lung, breast, colorectal, and other malignancies, underscoring their broad oncologic utility. In the setting of HPV-mediated oropharyngeal cancer, it offers highly sensitive and specific detection of viral tumor DNA for diagnosis, treatment response, and surveillance. Compared with traditional imaging and biopsy techniques, ctDNA provides a non-invasive, quantitative, and cost-effective means of monitoring MRD and predicting recurrence. Though it has limitations in early-stage disease, its detection threshold may precede radiographic confirmation by weeks to months, which may significantly alter receipt of timely therapy.

Integration of ctDNA into routine practice has the potential to improve outcomes by enabling earlier intervention, refining risk stratification, and reducing both direct and indirect healthcare costs. However, barriers to widespread implementation remain; inequitable access to testing, high assay costs, variability in detection methods, and limited long-term validation studies all contribute to the current lack of a standardized testing process and incorporation into clinical guidelines. As clinical trials and real-world evidence continue to mature, ctDNA holds promise as a transformative adjunct in cancer care. Accordingly, clinicians and researchers must remain cautiously optimistic, acknowledging that this is a rapidly developing field where clinical standards are likely to shift in the coming years.

Funding

None.

Conflicts of interest

None.

Author details

Mallory McKeon[1], Megha Mohanakrishnan[2], Priscilla F.A. Pichardo[1], Alice L. Tang[1], Chad A. Zender[1] and Dustin A. Silverman[1*]

1 Department of Otolaryngology, Head and Neck Surgery, University of Cincinnati Medical Center, Cincinnati, OH, USA

2 University of Cincinnati College of Medicine, Cincinnati, OH, USA

*Address all correspondence to: silverdt@ucmail.uc.edu

References

[1] Chow LQM. Head and neck cancer. The New England Journal of Medicine. 2020;**382**(1):60-72

[2] Goyal N, Day A, Epstein J, Goodman J, Graboyes E, Jalisi S, et al. Head and neck cancer survivorship consensus statement from the American Head and Neck Society. Laryngoscope Investigative Otolaryngology. 2022;**7**(1):70-92

[3] Bray F, Laversanne M, Sung H, Ferlay J, Siegel RL, Soerjomataram I, et al. Global cancer statistics 2022: GLOBOCAN estimates of incidence and mortality worldwide for 36 cancers in 185 countries. CA: A Cancer Journal for Clinicians. 2024;**74**(3):229-263

[4] Economopoulou P, de Bree R, Kotsantis I, Psyrri A. Diagnostic tumor markers in head and neck squamous cell carcinoma (HNSCC) in the clinical setting. Frontiers in Oncology. 2019;**9**:827

[5] Chaturvedi AK, Engels EA, Pfeiffer RM, Hernandez BY, Xiao W, Kim E, et al. Human papillomavirus and rising oropharyngeal cancer incidence in the United States. Journal of Clinical Oncology: Official Journal of the American Society of Clinical Oncology. 2011;**29**(32):4294-4301

[6] Blot WJ, McLaughlin JK, Winn DM, Austin DF, Greenberg RS, Preston-Martin S, et al. Smoking and drinking in relation to oral and pharyngeal cancer. Cancer Research. 1988;**48**(11):3282-3287

[7] Siegel RL, Kratzer TB, Giaquinto AN, Sung H, Jemal A. Cancer statistics, 2025. CA: A Cancer Journal for Clinicians. 2025;**75**(1):10-45

[8] Krane JF. Role of cytology in the diagnosis and management of HPV-associated head and neck carcinoma. Acta Cytologica. 2013;**57**(2):117-126

[9] Mehanna H, Beech T, Nicholson T, El-Hariry I, McConkey C, Paleri V, et al. Prevalence of human papillomavirus in oropharyngeal and nonoropharyngeal head and neck cancer--systematic review and meta-analysis of trends by time and region. Head & Neck. 2013;**35**(5):747-755

[10] Lechner M, Liu J, Masterson L, Fenton TR. HPV-associated oropharyngeal cancer: Epidemiology, molecular biology and clinical management. Nature Reviews. Clinical Oncology. 2022;**19**(5):306-327

[11] Taberna M, Mena M, Pavón MA, Alemany L, Gillison ML, Mesía R. Human papillomavirus-related oropharyngeal cancer. Annals of Oncology: Official Journal of the European Society for Medical Oncology. 2017;**28**(10):2386-2398

[12] Hafkamp HC, Manni JJ, Haesevoets A, Voogd AC, Schepers M, Bot FJ, et al. Marked differences in survival rate between smokers and nonsmokers with HPV 16-associated tonsillar carcinomas. International Journal of Cancer. 2008;**122**(12): 2656-2664

[13] Doorbar J, Quint W, Banks L, Bravo IG, Stoler M, Broker TR, et al. The biology and life-cycle of human papillomaviruses. Vaccine. 2012;**30**(Suppl. 5):F55-F70

[14] Huang X, Leo P, Jones L, Duijf PHG, Hartel G, Kenny L, et al. A comparison between mutational profiles in tumour tissue DNA and circulating tumour DNA in head and neck squamous

cell carcinoma - A systematic review. Mutation Research, Reviews in Mutation Research. 2024;**793**:108477

[15] Miller M, Shirole N, Tian R, Pal D, Sordella R. The evolution of TP53 mutations: From loss-of-function to separation-of-function mutants. Journal of Cancer Biology & Research. 2016;**4**(4):1091

[16] Seiwert TY, Zuo Z, Keck MK, Khattri A, Pedamallu CS, Stricker T, et al. Integrative and comparative genomic analysis of HPV-positive and HPV-negative head and neck squamous cell carcinomas. Clinical Cancer Research. 2015;**21**(3):632-641

[17] McKeon M, Gallant J-N, Kim Y, Das S. It takes two to tango: A review of oncogenic virus and host microbiome associated inflammation in head and neck cancer. Cancers. 2022;**14**(13):3120

[18] Riaz N, Morris LG, Lee W, Chan TA. Unraveling the molecular genetics of head and neck cancer through genome-wide approaches. Genes & Diseases. 2014;**1**(1):75-86

[19] Shaikh H, McGrath JE, Hughes B, Xiu J, Brodskiy P, Sukari A, et al. Genomic and molecular profiling of human papillomavirus associated head and neck squamous cell carcinoma treated with immune checkpoint blockade compared to survival outcomes. Cancers. 2021;**13**(24):6309

[20] Jakobsen KK, Bendtsen SK, Pallisgaard N, Friborg J, Lelkaitis G, Grønhøj C, et al. Liquid biopsies with circulating plasma HPV–DNA measurements—A clinically applicable surveillance tool for patients with HPV-positive oropharyngeal cancer. Clinical Cancer Research. 2023;**29**(19):3914-3923

[21] McLaughlin-Drubin ME, Münger K. The human papillomavirus E7 oncoprotein. Virology. 2009;**384**(2):335-344

[22] Vande Pol SB, Klingelhutz AJ. Papillomavirus E6 oncoproteins. Virology. 2013;**445**(1-2):115-137

[23] Ramqvist T, Mints M, Tertipis N, Näsman A, Romanitan M, Dalianis T. Studies on human papillomavirus (HPV) 16 E2, E5 and E7 mRNA in HPV-positive tonsillar and base of tongue cancer in relation to clinical outcome and immunological parameters. Oral Oncology. 2015;**51**(12):1126-1131

[24] Fakhry C, Gillison ML. Clinical implications of human papillomavirus in head and neck cancers. Journal of Clinical Oncology: Official Journal of the American Society of Clinical Oncology. 2006;**24**(17):2606-2611

[25] DeWeese TL, Walsh JC, Dillehay LE, Kessis TD, Hedrick L, Cho KR, et al. Human papillomavirus E6 and E7 oncoproteins alter cell cycle progression but not radiosensitivity of carcinoma cells treated with low-dose-rate radiation. International Journal of Radiation Oncology, Biology, Physics. 1997;**37**(1):145-154

[26] Siravegna G, O'Boyle CJ, Varmeh S, Queenan N, Michel A, Stein J, et al. Cell-free HPV DNA provides an accurate and rapid diagnosis of HPV-associated head and neck cancer. Clinical Cancer Research: An Official Journal of the American Association for Cancer Research. 2022;**28**(4):719-727

[27] Gillison ML, Alemany L, Snijders PJ, Chaturvedi A, Steinberg BM, Schwartz S, et al. Human papillomavirus and diseases of the upper airway: Head and neck cancer and respiratory papillomatosis. Vaccine. 2012;**30**(Suppl. 5):F34-F54

[28] Chen SY, Massa S, Mazul AL, Kallogjeri D, Yaeger L, Jackson RS,

et al. The association of smoking and outcomes in HPV-positive oropharyngeal cancer: A systematic review. American Journal of Otolaryngology. 2020;**41**(5):102592

[29] Kreimer AR, Clifford GM, Boyle P, Franceschi S. Human papillomavirus types in head and neck squamous cell carcinomas worldwide: A systematic review. Cancer Epidemiology, Biomarkers & Prevention: A Publication of the American Association for Cancer Research, cosponsored by the American Society of Preventive Oncology. 2005;**14**(2):467-475

[30] Ang KK, Harris J, Wheeler R, Weber R, Rosenthal DI, Nguyen-Tân PF, et al. Human papillomavirus and survival of patients with oropharyngeal cancer. The New England Journal of Medicine. 2010;**363**(1):24-35

[31] Guarino P, Chiari F, Cordeschi S, D'Alessio P, Ingelido C, Motta G, et al. A comprehensive systematic review on functional results, speech and swallowing outcomes after trans-Oral robotic surgery for oropharyngeal squamous cell cancer. Journal of Clinical Medicine. 2024;**13**(20):6039

[32] Golusinski P, Corry J, Poorten VV, Simo R, Sjögren E, Mäkitie A, et al. De-escalation studies in HPV-positive oropharyngeal cancer: How should we proceed? Oral Oncology. 2021;**123**:105620

[33] Adilbay D, Lele S, Pang J, Asarkar A, Calligas J, Nathan CA. Circulating human papillomavirus DNA in head and neck squamous cell carcinoma: Possible applications and future directions. Cancers. 2022;**14**(23):5946

[34] Hudečková M, Koucký V, Rottenberg J, Gál B. Gene mutations in circulating tumour DNA as a diagnostic and prognostic marker in head and neck cancer-a systematic review. Biomedicine. 2021;**9**(11):1548

[35] Wang Y, Springer S, Mulvey CL, Silliman N, Schaefer J, Sausen M, et al. Detection of somatic mutations and HPV in the saliva and plasma of patients with head and neck squamous cell carcinomas. Science Translational Medicine. 2015;**7**(293):293ra104

[36] Aulakh SS, Silverman DA, Young K, Dennis SK, Birkeland AC. The promise of circulating tumor DNA in head and neck cancer. Cancers. 2022;**14**(12):2968

[37] Ahn SM, Chan JYK, Zhang Z, Wang H, Khan Z, Bishop JA, et al. Saliva and plasma quantitative polymerase chain reaction–based detection and surveillance of human papillomavirus–related head and neck cancer. JAMA Otolaryngology–Head & Neck Surgery. 2014;**140**(9):846

[38] Galot R, Machiels J-PH. Current applications and challenges of circulating tumor DNA (ctDNA) in squamous cell carcinoma of the head and neck (SCCHN). Cancer Treatment Reviews. 2020;**85**:101992

[39] Naegele S, Ruiz-Torres DA, Zhao Y, Goss D, Faden DL. Comparing the diagnostic performance of quantitative PCR, digital droplet PCR, and next-generation sequencing liquid biopsies for human papillomavirus–associated cancers. The Journal of Molecular Diagnostics. 2024;**26**(3):179-190

[40] Adilbay D, Lele S, Pang J, Asarkar A, Calligas J, Nathan C-A. Circulating human papillomavirus DNA in head and neck squamous cell carcinoma: Possible applications and future directions. Cancers. 2022;**14**(23):5946

[41] Hanna GJ, Dennis MJ, Scarfo N, Mullin MS, Sethi RKV, Sehgal K, et al.

Personalized ctDNA for monitoring disease status in head and neck squamous cell carcinoma. Clinical Cancer Research. 2024;**30**(15):3329-3336

[42] Ferrandino RM, Chen S, Kappauf C, Barlow J, Gold BS, Berger MH, et al. Performance of liquid biopsy for diagnosis and surveillance of human papillomavirus–associated oropharyngeal cancer. JAMA Otolaryngology–Head & Neck Surgery. 2023;**149**(11):971

[43] Adelman AE, Motwani K, Chapurin N. Circulating tumor DNA testing for detection and surveillance of sinonasal HPV-associated cancers. Journal of Neurological Surgery Reports. 2025;**86**(2):e89-e91

[44] Karimi A, Jafari-Koshki T, Zehtabi M, Kargar F, Gheit T. Predictive impact of human papillomavirus circulating tumor DNA in treatment response monitoring of HPV-associated cancers; a meta-analysis on recurrent event endpoints. Cancer Medicine. 2023;**12**(17):17592-17602

[45] Lanman RB, Mortimer SA, Zill OA, Sebisanovic D, Lopez R, Blau S, et al. Analytical and clinical validation of a digital sequencing panel for quantitative, highly accurate evaluation of cell-free circulating tumor DNA. PLoS One. 2015;**10**(10):e0140712

[46] Chera BS, Kumar S, Shen C, Amdur R, Dagan R, Green R, et al. Plasma circulating tumor HPV DNA for the surveillance of cancer recurrence in HPV-associated oropharyngeal cancer. Journal of Clinical Oncology. 2020;**38**(10):1050-1058

[47] Yang Z, Gomez-Fernandez C, Lora Gonzalez M, Esebua M, Kerr DA. HPV testing through p16 immunocytochemistry in neck-mass FNA and its correlation with tissue samples. Cancer Cytopathology. 2019;**127**(7):458-464

[48] Chernesky M, Jang D, Schweizer J, Arias M, Doerwald-Munoz L, Gupta M, et al. HPV E6 oncoproteins and nucleic acids in neck lymph node fine needle aspirates and oral samples from patients with oropharyngeal squamous cell carcinoma. Papillomavirus Research. 2018;**6**:1-5

[49] Jakobsen KK, Carlander A-LF, Bendtsen SK, Garset-Zamani M, Lynggaard CD, Grønhøj C, et al. Diagnostic accuracy of HPV detection in patients with oropharyngeal squamous cell carcinomas: A systematic review and meta-analysis. Viruses. 2021;**13**(9):1692

[50] Rettig EM, Wang AA, Tran N-A, Carey E, Dey T, Schoenfeld JD, et al. Association of Pretreatment Circulating Tumor Tissue-Modified Viral HPV DNA with Clinicopathologic factors in HPV-positive oropharyngeal cancer. JAMA Otolaryngology – Head & Neck Surgery. 2022;**148**(12):1120-1130

[51] Cao Y, Haring CT, Brummel C, Bhambhani C, Aryal M, Lee C, et al. Early HPV ctDNA kinetics and imaging biomarkers predict therapeutic response in p16+ oropharyngeal squamous cell carcinoma. Clinical Cancer Research. 2022;**28**(2):350-359

[52] Chera BS, Kumar S, Beaty BT, Marron D, Jefferys S, Green R, et al. Rapid clearance profile of plasma circulating tumor HPV type 16 DNA during Chemoradiotherapy correlates with disease control in HPV-associated oropharyngeal cancer. Clinical Cancer Research: An Official Journal of the American Association for Cancer Research. 2019;**25**(15):4682-4690

[53] Hanna GJ, Supplee JG, Kuang Y, Mahmood U, Lau CJ, Haddad RI, et al.

Plasma HPV cell-free DNA monitoring in advanced HPV-associated oropharyngeal cancer. Annals of Oncology. 2018;**29**(9): 1980-1986

[54] Kumari S, Mishra S, Ali W. Circulating biomarkers in HPV-associated oropharyngeal cancer: Clinical applications of liquid biopsy in diagnosis, prognosis, and surveillance. The Journal of Liquid Biopsy. 2025;**9**:100316

[55] Carron R, Gaudy-Marqueste C, Amatore F, Padovani L, Malissen N, Balossier A, et al. Stereotactic radiosurgery combined with anti-PD1 for the management of melanoma brain metastases: A retrospective study of safety and efficacy. European Journal of Cancer. 2020;**135**:52-61

[56] Huttinger ZM, Gogineni E, Baliga S, Blakaj DM, Bhateja P, Bonomi M, et al. Circulating tumor DNA determines induction chemotherapy response in HPV associated oropharyngeal squamous cell carcinoma: A pilot study. Oral Oncology. 2025;**161**:107179

[57] Yin LX, Hidalgo CM, Bogan AW, Hunter DE, Bartemes KR, Tasche KK, et al. Postoperative ctHPVDNA kineticsin patients with HPV-related oropharyngeal cancer. JAMA Otolaryngology–Head & Neck Surgery. 14 May 2025:e251606. DOI: 10.1001/jamaoto.2025.1606. Epub ahead of print

[58] Efthymiou V, Queenan N, Haas M, Naegele S, Goss D, Faden DL. Circulating tumor DNA in the immediate postoperative setting. Annals of Surgical Oncology. 2024;**31**(4):2319-2325

[59] Berger BM, Hanna GJ, Posner MR, Genden EM, Lautersztain J, Naber SP, et al. Detection of occult recurrence using circulating tumor tissue modified viral HPV DNA among patients treated for HPV-driven oropharyngeal carcinoma. Clinical Cancer Research. 2022;**28**(19):4292-4301

[60] Hanna GJ, Lau CJ, Mahmood U, Supplee JG, Mogili AR, Haddad RI, et al. Salivary HPV DNA informs locoregional disease status in advanced HPV-associated oropharyngeal cancer. Oral Oncology. 2019;**95**:120-126

[61] Rettig EM, Faden DL, Sandhu S, Wong K, Faquin WC, Warinner C, et al. Detection of circulating tumor human papillomavirus DNA before diagnosis of HPV-positive head and neck cancer. International Journal of Cancer. 2022;**151**(7):1081-1085

[62] Campo F, Iocca O, Paolini F, Manciocco V, Moretto S, De Virgilio A, et al. The landscape of circulating tumor HPV DNA and TTMV-HPVDNA for surveillance of HPV-oropharyngeal carcinoma: Systematic review and meta-analysis. Journal of Experimental & Clinical Cancer Research. 2024;**43**(1):215

[63] Kais A, Santiago SP, Han PC, Clump DA, Stokes WA, Fancy T, et al. Human papillomavirus circulating tumor DNA: A diagnostic tool in squamous cell carcinoma of unknown primary—A pilot study. Frontiers in Oncology. 2024;**14**:1376595

[64] Chen L, Cohen M, Hatzoglou V, Zhang Z, Riaz N, Wong RJ, et al. Early disease recurrence following post-operative HPV ctDNA directed active surveillance in oropharyngeal carcinoma – Outcomes of a prospective pilot study. International Journal of Radiation Oncology*Biology*Physics. 2024;**118**(5):e91

[65] Braig F, Voigtlaender M, Schieferdecker A, Busch C-J, Laban S, Grob T, et al. Liquid biopsy monitoring uncovers acquired RAS-mediated resistance to cetuximab in a substantial

proportion of patients with head and neck squamous cell carcinoma. Oncotarget. 2016;7(28):42988-42995

[66] Di Nicolantonio F, Martini M, Molinari F, Sartore-Bianchi A, Arena S, Saletti P, et al. Wild-type *BRAF* is required for response to Panitumumab or Cetuximab in metastatic colorectal cancer. Journal of Clinical Oncology. 2008;**26**(35):5705-5712

[67] Dasari A, Morris VK, Allegra CJ, Atreya C, Benson AB, Boland P, et al. ctDNA applications and integration in colorectal cancer: An NCI colon and rectal–anal task forces whitepaper. Nature Reviews Clinical Oncology. 2020;**17**(12):757-770

[68] Lewis JS, Beadle B, Bishop JA, Chernock RD, Colasacco C, Kalicanin T, et al. Human papillomavirus testing in head and neck carcinomas: Guideline update. Archives of Pathology & Laboratory Medicine. 2025;**149**(6):e115-ee50

[69] Maghami E, Ismaila N, Alvarez A, Chernock R, Duvvuri U, Geiger J, et al. Diagnosis and Management of Squamous Cell Carcinoma of unknown primary in the head and neck: ASCO guideline. Journal of Clinical Oncology. 2020;**38**(22):2570-2596

[70] Siravegna G, Marsoni S, Siena S, Bardelli A. Integrating liquid biopsies into the management of cancer. Nature Reviews Clinical Oncology. 2017;**14**(9):531-548

[71] Kowalchuk RO, Kamdem Talom BC, Van Abel KM, Ma DM, Waddle MR, Routman DM. Estimated cost of circulating tumor DNA for Posttreatment surveillance of human papillomavirus–associated oropharyngeal cancer. JAMA Network Open. 2022;**5**(1):e2144783

[72] Araujo M, Bouassaly J, Farshadi F, Hier M, Mascarella M, Mlynarek A, et al. Current status of circulating tumor DNA and circulating cell alterations in HPV-associated head and neck cancer. Oral Oncology. 2025;**167**:107417

[73] Rosi-Schumacher M, Patel S, Phan C, Goyal N. Understanding financial toxicity in patients with head and neck cancer: A systematic review. Clinical Medicine Insights Oncology. 2023;**17**:11795549221147730

Section 2

Therapeutic Updates

Chapter 3

Chemoradiation for HPV-Negative Oropharyngeal Cancer: What Have We Achieved?

Trinanjan Basu, Rohith R. Menon, Jay P. Sahu and Ghazala K. Roshan

Abstract

Oropharyngeal squamous cell carcinoma (OPSCC) represents a challenging and biologically diverse disease within the spectrum of head and neck malignancies. The treatment landscape over the past two to three decades has been significantly altered by the human papillomavirus (HPV) association. Whereas HPV+ OPSCC remains a biologically favorable cohort, the HPV represents a challenge, especially in developing nations due to the preponderance of tobacco association and inherent poor biology leading to dismal outcome. This chapter will address the biology of HPV-OPSCC, available treatment paradigms and outcomes, treatment scheme as of today and what future holds in treatment decisions. We also will highlight specific studies and data related to the Indian scenario.

Keywords: HPV, oropharyngeal cancer, outcome, future direction, Indian data

1. Introduction

Oropharyngeal squamous cell carcinoma (OPSCC) represents a challenging and biologically diverse disease within the spectrum of head and neck malignancies. Over the past two to three decades, the landscape of OPSCC management has been significantly altered by the discovery and clinical validation of human papillomavirus (HPV) as a major etiological agent in a subset of cases. This pivotal finding led to a shift in our understanding of OPSCC, which is now broadly categorized into two distinct entities: HPV-associated (p16-positive) and HPV-negative (p16-negative) cancers [1, 2]. HPV-positive tumors, most commonly linked to HPV-16, typically affect younger patients, often without a history of tobacco or alcohol use. These cancers exhibit a favorable biology marked by high radiosensitivity and robust immune responsiveness and are associated with significantly improved outcomes [3, 4]. The growing recognition that HPV-associated oropharyngeal squamous cell carcinoma (OPSCC) represents a distinct clinical and biological entity, coupled with an increased understanding of the detrimental effects of conventional treatments on speech, swallowing, taste, and overall psychosocial well-being, has generated considerable multidisciplinary interest in tailoring treatment strategies based on HPV status. Despite this distinction, current therapeutic guidelines for HPV-positive and HPV-negative OPSCC remain largely uniform, pending the results of ongoing clinical trials aimed at refining risk stratification and personalizing management. Given the oropharynx's pivotal role in functions such as articulation and deglutition, the treatment of tumors in this region can have profound implications on patients' post-treatment quality of life [5]. As such, therapeutic approaches must strive to maintain high cure rates while simultaneously minimizing long-term functional morbidity. Advances in this domain have facilitated the emergence of de-escalation protocols, biomarker-guided therapy and ongoing efforts to reduce treatment-related toxicity while maintaining excellent oncologic control [6]. In stark contrast, HPV-negative OPSCC, often defined by the absence of p16 overexpression, remains a formidable therapeutic challenge. These tumors tend to occur in older patients with significant exposure to traditional carcinogens such as tobacco and alcohol, and they follow a more aggressive clinical trajectory. Despite the use of modern radiotherapy techniques and concurrent systemic therapy, outcomes remain suboptimal with the high rates of recurrence, distant failure and reduced overall survival [7]. Epidemiologically, the burden of p16-negative OPSCC remains disproportionately high in low- and middle-income countries (LMICs) where tobacco consumption, both smoked and smokeless and alcohol use are endemic [8]. In such regions, HPV-negative cancers remain the dominant subtype. Unfortunately, this group of patients are significantly under-represented in clinical trials leading to a therapeutic framework largely borrowed from HPV-positive population and this has created a significant translational and therapeutic gap.

Concurrent chemoradiotherapy (CRT) continues to be the cornerstone of non-surgical management for locally advanced OPSCC. However, the landmark clinical trials that inform modern CRT protocols such as RTOG 0129 and 0522 did not stratify or power their analyses based on HPV status [9, 10]. As a result, the applicability of their findings to p16-negative disease is questionable. In clinical practice, we continue to treat HPV-negative patients with regimens optimized for HPV-positive disease despite their distinct biology and inferior outcomes [11]. Over the years, multiple strategies have been explored to improve outcomes in p16-negative OPSCC. Yet, these efforts have largely failed to demonstrate consistent, practice-changing results. With this background, a pressing question emerges: Have we truly made any progress in treating p16-negative OPSCC, or are we witnessing a state of therapeutic inertia?

This manuscript aims to address that question by revisiting the underlying biology of p16-negative disease, summarizing current evidence on CRT outcomes and highlighting avenues for future therapeutic development. The goal is to stimulate critical thinking and re-evaluate how we approach this high-risk, underserved patient population.

2. Biology and prognostic implications of p16-negative OPSCC

Biologically, p16-negative OPSCC is a distinct clinical entity that differs markedly from HPV-associated tumors in terms of pathogenesis, molecular profile, and treatment response [12]. These cancers are often keratinizing, poorly differentiated and linked to chronic exposure to environmental carcinogens, most notably tobacco and alcohol. This carcinogenic exposure leads to a field cancerization effect which predisposes to multifocal tumor development, synchronous primaries, and resistance to conventional therapy [13]. At the molecular level, p16-negative tumors are characterized by frequent TP53 mutations, loss of CDKN2A, and amplification of EGFR, among other alterations [14]. This has been shown in **Figure 1**.

The oncogenic mechanisms of HPV E6 and E7 oncoproteins play a critical role in promoting malignant transformation by disrupting key regulatory pathways of the cell cycle, apoptosis, and genomic stability. E7 helps break down a key cell cycle regulator called pRb using a special complex, pushing cells to divide uncontrollably. It also blocks p21, which normally stops the cell cycle, allowing abnormal cell growth. E6 breaks down the p53 protein, which is vital for repairing DNA and causing damaged cells to die, so cells survive even with genetic damage. As pRb is lost, a feedback loop increases p16 levels, which normally stop cell growth, but the pathway is bypassed. These genetic abnormalities disrupt cell cycle control, inhibit apoptotic signaling, and impair DNA repair mechanisms, contributing to uncontrolled growth, treatment resistance, and aggressive behavior [11]. Importantly, the tumor microenvironment of p16-negative OPSCC is typically hypoxic, fibrotic, and immunosuppressive. These "immune-cold" tumors are poorly infiltrated by effector immune cells such as CD8+ cytotoxic T-lymphocytes, and they show limited response to immunotherapeutic agents [15]. This contrasts with HPV-positive cancers that are more immunogenic and display higher levels of immune activation. Histologically, p16-negative OPSCCs are more likely to present with high-risk features, including perineural invasion, lymphovascular emboli, and extracapsular spread in lymph nodes. These adverse pathological features further contribute to the high incidence of locoregional failure and distant metastasis. Moreover, p16-negative tumors often arise in a multifocal and metachronous manner, complicating both surveillance and salvage strategies. Clinically, the impact of these biological differences is profound. Numerous studies have demonstrated that p16-negative OPSCC is associated with significantly worse overall survival (OS) and disease-free survival

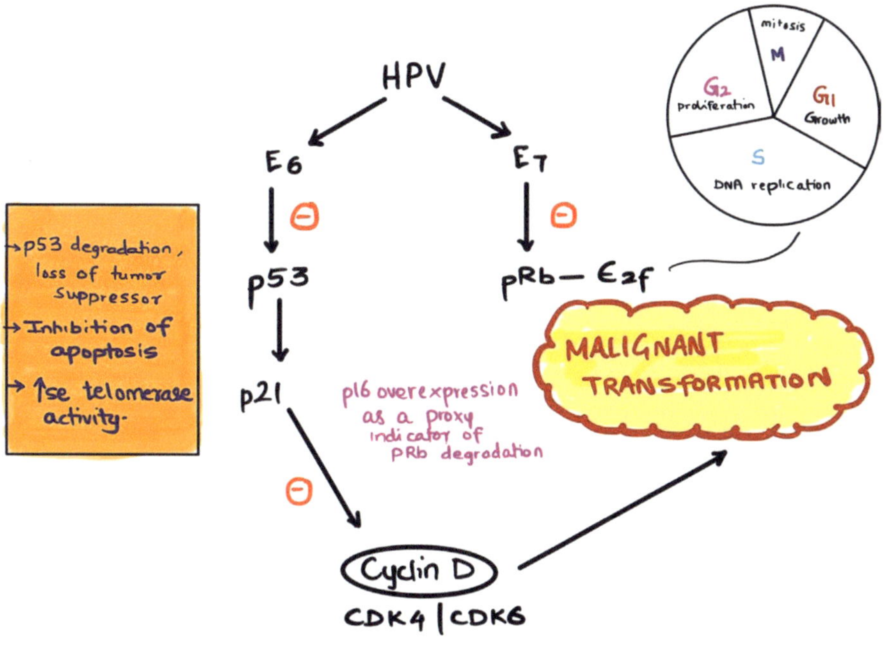

Figure 1.
Biology and carcinogenesis of HPV.

(DFS) compared to HPV-positive disease, even when treated with high-quality intensity-modulated radiotherapy (IMRT) and concurrent cisplatin. Unlike their HPV-positive counterparts, these patients do not benefit from treatment de-intensification and, in many cases, may require treatment intensification to achieve acceptable control [16]. Despite these challenges, CRT remains the current standard of care. The addition of high-dose cisplatin to radiotherapy has shown the modest survival benefit in p16-negative disease, though toxicity remains a significant barrier to completion.

3. Literature on outcome

RTOG 9003 phase III trial (International Journal of Radiation Oncology Biology Physics, 2000) compared standard fractionation radiotherapy (70 Gy in 35 fractions over 7 weeks) to three altered fractionation regimens hyperfractionation (81.6 Gy in 68 twice-daily fractions), accelerated fractionation with split (67.2 Gy in 42 fractions), and accelerated fractionation continuous (72 Gy in 42 fractions) in patients with locally advanced head and neck squamous cell carcinoma. A total of 1113 patients randomized across the four arms showed significantly higher LRC with hyperfractionation ($p = 0.045$) and continuous accelerated fractionation ($p = 0.050$) compared to standard fractionation along with improved DFS. Acute grade 3–4 mucositis greater with altered fractionation arms compared to conventional. The study concluded that hyperfractionation improved LRC [17].

The Adelstein et al. Intergroup phase III trial (Journal of Clinical Oncology, 2003) compared standard radiotherapy alone versus two schedules of concurrent chemoradiotherapy in 321 patients with unresectable HNSCC, who received either radiation alone or radiation plus high-dose cisplatin every 3 weeks, or radiation plus low-dose weekly cisplatin. The primary outcome, OS, significantly improved in the high-dose cisplatin arm compared to radiation alone. Acute reactions were higher in both CRT arms [18].

The DAHANCA 6 & 7 randomized controlled trial (The Lancet, 2003) evaluated if accelerating radiotherapy by delivering six fractions per week improved outcomes compared to five fractions per week. A total of 1483 patients randomized to receive conventional radiotherapy (66–68 Gy in 33–34 fractions) over 5 versus 6 fractions per week, shortening treatment duration by 1 week in the accelerated arm. Accelerated treatment significantly improved LRC (64% vs. 76% at 5 years; $p = 0.0001$) and disease-specific survival (66% vs. 73%). Acute mucositis grade 3–4 was higher with six fractions [19].

The GORTEC 94–01 trial (*Journal of Clinical Oncology*, 2004) compared radiotherapy alone with concurrent chemoradiotherapy in patients with stage III–IV oropharyngeal squamous cell carcinoma. A total of 226 patients were randomized to receive either radiotherapy alone (70 Gy in 35 fractions) or radiotherapy plus concurrent carboplatin (70 mg/m^2 days 1–4) and 5-fluorouracil (600 mg/m^2 days 1–4) for three cycles. At 5 years, OS was significantly higher in the chemoradiotherapy arm, and LRC was nearly doubled. Mucositis (grade 3–4) increased with chemoradiotherapy [20].

The comparative analysis by Bernier et al. (Head & Neck, 2005) examined outcomes from the EORTC 22931 and RTOG 9501 trials to better define risk groups in patients receiving postoperative chemoradiotherapy for locally advanced head and neck squamous cell carcinoma. The pooled analysis of both trials showed that adding cisplatin-based chemotherapy significantly improved LRC and DFS in patients with positive margins and extracapsular nodal extension [21].

The MARCH meta-analysis (The Lancet, 2006) by Bourhis et al. pooled data from 15 randomized trials including 6515 patients to assess whether altered fractionation radiotherapy (hyperfractionation or accelerated fractionation) improved OS compared to conventional radiotherapy. Hyperfractionation significantly improved OS (8% absolute survival benefit at 5 years), while accelerated fractionation with and without total dose reduction showed a smaller benefit (2% and 1.7%). LRC improved with hyperfractionation (6.4% at 5 years). Effect more pronounced in younger patients.(<50 yrs). Acute grade 3–4 mucositis was higher in altered fractionation arms (58% vs. 34%) [22].

The MACH-NC meta-analysis update (Radiotherapy and Oncology, 2009) by Pignon et al. assessed the impact of chemotherapy added to locoregional treatment in head and neck squamous cell carcinoma by pooling data from 87 randomized trials including 16,485 patients. The addition of chemotherapy provided a significant OS benefit, with an absolute survival improvement of 4.5% at 5 years (hazard ratio 0.88, $p < 0.0001$). The benefit was greatest when chemotherapy was administered concurrently with radiotherapy (hazard ratio 0.81), leading to a 6.5% absolute survival gain at 5 years. Platinum-based regimens are preferred [11].

The TAX 324 randomized phase 3 trial (The Lancet Oncology, 2011) compared induction chemotherapy with cisplatin and fluorouracil (PF) versus docetaxel, cisplatin, and fluorouracil (TPF) followed by chemoradiotherapy in patients with locally advanced squamous cell carcinoma. A total of 501 patients were randomized to receive either 3 cycles of PF (cisplatin 100 mg/m^2 + fluorouracil 1000 mg/m^2/day ×5 days) or three cycles of TPF (docetaxel 75 mg/m^2 day 1, cisplatin 100 mg/m^2 day 1, fluorouracil 1000 mg/m^2/day ×4 days) before radiotherapy with weekly carboplatin. Mean OS was significantly improved in the TPF arm (70.6 months vs. 34.8%). PFS was also better in the TPF arm [23].

The RTOG 9501/Intergroup phase III trial (Journal of Clinical Oncology, 2012) assessed whether postoperative radiotherapy plus concurrent cisplatin chemotherapy improved outcomes compared to radiotherapy alone in patients with high-risk resected head and neck squamous cell carcinoma. A total of 410 patients randomized to receive radiotherapy (60–66 Gy) alone or combined with cisplatin 100 mg/m^2 on days 1, 22, and 43. After median 10.1 years of follow-up, LRC remained improved in the chemoradiotherapy group, although overall survival was similar. Subset analysis in patients with positive margins or extracapsular nodal extension showed improved OS (19.6 vs. 27.1%), grade 3–4 acute toxicities occurred chemoradiation patients [24].

The GORTEC 99–02 trial (The Lancet, 2012) was an open-label, phase 3 study comparing standard chemoradiotherapy, accelerated radiotherapy alone, and accelerated radiotherapy with concomitant chemotherapy in patients with locally advanced carcinoma. A total of 840 patients were randomized to receive either standard radiotherapy with three cycles of cisplatin 100 mg/m^2, accelerated radiotherapy alone (70 Gy over 6 weeks with 6 fractions/week), or accelerated radiotherapy with cisplatin. At 3 years, PFS was significantly better with standard chemoradiotherapy followed by accelerated chemoradiotherapy followed by radiotherapy alone. Grade 3–4 mucositis occurred in accelerated radiotherapy alone [25].

The PARADIGM trial (Journal of Clinical Oncology, 2013) was a randomized phase 3 study comparing sequential therapy (induction chemotherapy followed by concurrent chemoradiotherapy) with concurrent chemoradiotherapy alone in patients with locally advanced head and neck squamous cell carcinoma. A total of 145 patients were randomized to receive three cycles of TPF induction chemotherapy (docetaxel 75 mg/m^2, cisplatin 75 mg/m^2, fluorouracil 750 mg/m^2/day ×5 days) followed by chemoradiation, or chemoradiation alone with cisplatin (100 mg/m^2 every 3 weeks). At 3 years, OS was not significantly different (73% with induction vs. 78% without; hazard ratio 1.09; p = 0.74) and PFS also similar. Grade 3–4 neutropenia was greater in the induction group [26].

The phase III trial by Cohen et al. (Journal of Clinical Oncology, 2014) evaluated whether induction chemotherapy improved outcomes before chemoradiotherapy in patients with N2 or N3 locally advanced head and neck squamous cell carcinoma. A total of 285 patients were randomized to receive either induction chemotherapy with paclitaxel, cisplatin, and fluorouracil for three cycles followed by concurrent chemoradiotherapy, or concurrent chemoradiotherapy alone. The primary endpoint, OS, showed no significant difference at 3 years [27].

The RTOG 0522 trial (Journal of Clinical Oncology, 2014), randomized phase III study evaluating if adding cetuximab (anti-EGFR) to accelerated radiotherapy plus high-dose cisplatin improved outcomes in stage III–IV carcinoma. A total of 891 patients were randomized to receive accelerated radiation (72 Gy in 42 fractions over 6 weeks) plus cisplatin (100 mg/m^2 on days 1 and 22) with or without cetuximab (400 mg/m^2 loading dose, then 250 mg/m^2 weekly). Adding cetuximab did not improve PFS/OS and overall disease control grade ≥ 3 mucositis (43.2%) and acneiform rash (25%) were seen in cetuximab-treated patients. PFS and OS were higher in patients with p16-positive OPC. Outcomes did not differ by EGFR expression [10].

The ORATOR trial (The Lancet Oncology, 2019) was an open-label, phase 2 randomized study comparing primary radiotherapy/chemoradiation versus transoral robotic surgery (TORS) with neck dissection in patients with early-stage (T1–T2, N0–2) oropharyngeal squamous cell carcinoma. Sixty-eight patients were enrolled. At 1 year, the swallowing-related quality of life (MDADI score) was slightly better in the radiotherapy group (mean score 86.9 vs. 80.1, p = 0.042 [28]).

The KEYNOTE-412 study (Lancet Oncology, 2024) was a phase 3 trial that enrolled 402 patients with locally advanced carcinoma to evaluate whether adding pembrolizumab to standard chemoradiotherapy would improve outcomes. Patients were randomized to receive either 14 cycles of 200 mg pembrolizumab (one cycle prior to CRT, every 3 weeks induction and maintenance 200 mg every 3 weeks) or placebo. The primary endpoint, median event-free survival 71.8 months vs. 49.8 months, showed a hazard ratio of 0.80, p = 0.043 with pembrolizumab. No OS benefit was observed [29].

JAVELIN trial (Lancet Oncology, 2021) randomized, double-blind, placebo-controlled, phase 3 trial evaluating avelumab plus standard chemoradiotherapy (CRT) versus CRT alone in patients with locally advanced carcinoma. A total of 697 patients were randomly assigned to receive either avelumab (10 mg/kg every 2 weeks) with CRT or placebo with CRT. Adding avelumab did not significantly improve PFS, with a median follow-up for PFS of 14.6 months in the avelumab group versus 14.8 months in the placebo group. Median PFS was not reached [30].

Nimotuzumab in Head and Neck Cancer was a phase 3, randomized trial including 536 patients with locally advanced squamous cell carcinoma to receive either radical radiotherapy (66–70 Gy) with concurrent weekly cisplatin (30 mg/m^2) (CRT) or CRT with weekly nimotuzumab (200 mg) (NCRT). The primary endpoint (PFS) was improved (HR-0.69, p = .004), and secondary endpoints were DFS, LRC, and OS, showing a trend toward improvement. Grade 3 mucositis was higher in the NCRT arm (66.7 vs. 55.8%) [31].

Al-Mamgani et al. conducted a matched-pair analysis comparing toxicity and outcomes of IMRT versus 3DCRT in 92 matched patients each with oropharyngeal cancer

Trial	Inclusion/ Exclusion	Comparison arms	Primary endpoint	Key outcomes	Conclusion
RTOG 9003 (2000) [17]	Stage III–IV HNSCC Oropharynx-649	Standard RT vs. Hyperfractionation vs. Accelerated RT with split vs. Accelerated fractionation with boost	Locoregional Control (LRC)	Better LRC-Hyperfractionation and accelerated RT with concomitant boost; similar OS; ↑ mucositis in altered RT	Altered RT improves LRC
Adelstein et al. [18]	Unresectable HNSCC Oral cavity-36 Oropharynx-110 Hypopharynx-50 Larynx-25	Arm A-RT Arm B CRT days 1,22, 43 bolus cisplatin Arm C CRT 3 weekly FU+ bolus cisplatin	Overall Survival (OS)	Median OS: Arm A-12.6 mo Arm B-19.1 mo (p-0.014) Arm C-midway ↑ mucositis with CRT	CRT with cisplatin becomes standard
DAHANCA 6&7 (2003) [19]	T1–T4a, N0–N2b HNSCC; Pharynx-435	RT 5fr/week vs. 6fr/week (same dose)	LRC	5-yr LRC: 64% vs. 76%; DSS 66% vs. 73%; p = 0.0001	Moderate acceleration improves control
GORTEC 94–01 (2004) [20]	Stage III–IV OPSCC Oropharynx-226	RT vs. CRT (carboplatin +5FU)	OS	OS: 22.4% vs. 16%; DFS-27% vs. 15%, LRC: 48% vs. 25%; ↑ mucositis in CRT	CRT improves OS and LRC
MARCH Metalysis (2006) [22]	6515 pts. from 15 RCTs Oropharynx + larynx 5221	Hyper/Accelerated RT vs. Standard RT	OS	OS benefit with hyperfractionation 8% at 5 years (HR-0.92) Accelerated RT-2% at 5 years LRC ↑	Hyperfractionation has the greatest benefit on OS.
MACH-NC (2009) [11]	17,346 pts. from 93 RCTs Oropharynx-2349	RT ± Chemo (adjuvant, induction, concurrent)	OS	OS benefit at 5 years: +4.5% (concurrent CRT: +6.5%)	Concurrent CRT is most effective
GORTEC 9902 (2012) [25]	LA-HNSCC Oropharynx-555	Arm A-CRT Arm B-Accelerated CRT Arm C-Accelerated RT	PFS	3 yr. PFS 37.6%; 34.1%; 32.2% Accelerated RT had higher mucositis.	Chemotherapy has treatment effect that is not replaceable by accelerated RT.

Trial	Inclusion/ Exclusion	Comparison arms	Primary endpoint	Key outcomes	Conclusion
RTOG 0522 (2014) [10]	Stage III–IV HNSCC P16 positive-235 P16 negative-86	Arm A-CRT (cisplatin) Arm B-CRT (cisplatin) + cetuximab	PFS	No PFS /OS difference Arm A-61.2% /72.9% Arm B-58.9%/75.8% HR-0.93, p-0.49 Grade 3 /4 toxicity ↑ with cetuximab. P16+ responded better	Cetuximab is not beneficial in CRT
ORATOR (2019 &2024) [28]	T1–T2, N0–2 OPSCC n-68	CRT vs. TORS + ND	Swallow QoL (MDADI) EORTC QLQ-C30 and H&N35 scores	At 2 years, MDADI is better with RT (86.9 vs. 80.1); OS similar	Function preservation is better with RT. Disease control is excellent with either modality.
KEYNOTE-412 (2024) [29]	LA-HNSCC oropharynx- p16 negative T1-T4 N2a-3 p16 positive T4 or N3	CRT ± pembrolizumab	Event-Free Survival (EFS)	Median EFS-71.8 vs. 49.8 mo OS-NR	Pembrolizumab-not practice changing.
JAVELIN TRIAL [30]	HN SCC Oropharynx-326	CRT+/− Avelumab	PFS	NR Treatment-related adverse events	Safety profile needs to be evaluated. Currently, not the treatment of choice

Table 1.
Global data on key trials in HPV-OPSCC.

from a prospectively maintained institutional registry. IMRT significantly reduced grade 3 acute toxicity and tube feeding requirement, late dysphagia (10 vs. 31%, p = 0.004) and xerostomia (13 vs. 37%, p = 0.001). LRC, DFS, and OS were similar. IMRT offers a superior therapeutic ratio by significantly reducing treatment-related toxicity without compromising oncologic outcome [32].

Trial	Inclusion/ Exclusion	Comparison arms	Primary endpoint	Key outcomes	Conclusion
RTOG 9501 (update 2012) [21]	Post-op HNSCC Total n-410	RT vs. CRT	LRC	LRC ↑ with CRT Locoregional failures- RT-28.8% CRT-22.3% PFS, OS-similar; ↑ toxicity	CRT for positive margins/ENE.
Bernier et al. [21]	High-risk post-op HNSCC Oropharynx EORTC 22931–30% RTOG 9501–42%	Comparative analysis of EORTC 22931 & RTOG 9501	PFS	Greatest benefit in positive margins/ENE positive. EORTC 22931- PFS: 47% vs. 36%; OS: 53% vs. 40%; ↑ toxicity in CRT	CRT for select high-risk pts. only

Table 2.
Postoperative chemoradiation trials.

Trial	Inclusion/ Exclusion	Comparison arms	Primary endpoint	Key outcomes	Conclusion
TAX 324 [23]	LA-HNSCC Oropharynx – 80	TPF vs. PF → CRT	OS	5 yr. OS: 52% vs. 42% Median OS-70.6 mo vs. 34.8 mo. Tube dependency is greater in the PF arm	TPF is superior to PF
PARADIGM [26]	LA-HNSCC Oropharynx-80	TPF → CRT vs. CRT	OS	No OS difference(78% vs. 73%) HR-1.09; ↑ toxicity with induction	Induction chemo is recommended for select high-risk cases
Cohen et al. [27]	N2/N3 HNSCC Oropharynx-159	TPF → CRT vs. CRT	OS	OS- No significant difference. (HR-0.91) Decrease in metastasis.	Induction adds toxicity, not OS

Table 3.
Induction chemotherapy trials.

Trial	Inclusion	Comparison arms	Primary endpoint	Key outcomes	Status/ Conclusion
Definitive CTRT with IMRT using SIB in major p16 negative cohort [7]	ve Stage III-IV OPSCC p16 positive- 20 p16 negative- 49 not tested- 46	Single arm CTRT + SIB	2 year DFS	OS, QoL, Toxicity	P16 negative- 47% P16 positive- 83% Ongoing; aims to guide HPV-ve treatment in India
Nimotuzu m ab in Head and Neck Cancer [31]	LA HNSCC Oropharynx P16 positive-24 P16 negative-187	CRT+/- Nimotuzumab	PFS	2 yr PFS-61.8% vs 50.1 % HR-0.69	Novel alternative therapeutic option.

Table 4.
Indian data on HPV OPSCC.

The details of global data, postoperative chemoradiation and Indian data have been enumerated in **Tables 1–4**.

4. Overall treatment scheme

1. T1–T2N0 (Stage I, II)

   Treatment of choice: Definitive radiotherapy alone in a dose of 66–70 Gy in 33–35 fractions over 6.5 to 7 weeks.
   Alternative: Surgery (Transoral robotic surgery/Transoral laser microsurgery).
   Adjuvant treatment: Radiotherapy is indicated if the postsurgical histopathology report is suggestive of pT3/T4, close margins, multiple lymph nodes positive, neck nodes II-IV positive, perineural invasion, or lymphovascular invasion. Adjuvant chemoradiation (CRT) is indicated for positive margins and positive extranodal extension. Adjuvant radiotherapy is delivered in a dose of 60 Gy in 30 fractions over 6 weeks, along with weekly concurrent cisplatin (30 mg/m^2).

2. T1-T2N1, T3-T4N0-2c (Stage III, IVa)

   Treatment of choice: Definitive chemoradiation along with simultaneous integrated boost (SIB) to nodes. Radiotherapy dose and fractionation remain the same. Concurrent cisplatin (30 mg/m^2) weekly or 3 weekly (100 mg/m^2 x 3 cycles to be administered. For cisplatin-ineligible candidates, weekly nimotuzumab (200 mg) can be considered or altered fractionation radiotherapy.
   Alternative: Surgical resection of the primary along with ipsilateral/bilateral neck dissection.
   Adjuvant treatment: Same as Stage I, II

3. T4b Any N, AnyTN3 (Stage IVB)

Induction chemotherapy with three cycles of the TPF regimen followed by chemoradiation. Consider adding nimotuzumab or cetuximab to CRT.

4. Recurrent/Metastatic setting:

Systemic therapy: Pembrolizumab monotherapy or pembrolizumab + platin+5 FU.
Palliative radiotherapy for symptomatic control.

5. Future developments and scope in p16-negative oropharyngeal squamous cell carcinoma

As the current treatment paradigms are largely based on cisplatin-based chemoradiation, which have reached a therapeutic plateau, future strategies aim to integrate molecular profiling, targeted therapies, immunotherapy, and refined radiation delivery to improve the outcomes.

5.1 Refining diagnostic precision in HPV-negative OPSCC

There exists notable discordance between p16 immunohistochemistry and actual HPV status, with some tumors being p16-negative yet HPV-positive or vice versa. Future advances must prioritize precise discrimination between truly HPV-negative tumors and those falsely classified based on p16 immunohistochemistry alone. Incorporation of HPV E6/E7 mRNA-based assays, which confirm active viral oncogene transcription, offers a biologically meaningful improvement over a surrogate marker like p16. Integrating these assays with current diagnostics can refine staging, prevent inappropriate treatment de-escalation, and enhance stratification in clinical trials [33].

5.2 Molecular stratification and biomarker integration

With the advent of molecular profiling, efforts are underway to identify clinically actionable subtypes within this group. One of the most promising findings is MGMT (O6-methylguanine-DNA methyltransferase) promoter hypermethylation, which silences the MGMT gene: a critical DNA repair enzyme that removes alkyl adducts from the O6 position of guanine. When MGMT is silenced, tumor cells become less capable of repairing DNA damage caused by radiation or alkylating agents, potentially enhancing treatment response. A study by Jensen et al. showed improved local control in p16-negative OPSCC patients with MGMT hypermethylation after radiotherapy [34]. If validated in larger cohorts, MGMT methylation testing could serve as both a prognostic and predictive biomarker, guiding treatment intensification or inclusion of alkylating chemotherapy.

5.3 Breaking the cycle: To overcome radioresistance in p16-negative OPSCC

Adavosertib (AZD1775) is a WEE1 kinase inhibitor that disrupts the G2/M checkpoint, forcing damaged tumor cells into mitotic catastrophe. In p16-negative OPSCC, where TP53 mutations are common and G1 checkpoint control is lost, WEE1 inhibition selectively enhances radiosensitivity and cytotoxicity. The early phase I WISTERIA trial has demonstrated promising efficacy when combined with chemoradiation, especially in TP53-mutated or genomically unstable tumors [35]. As a strategy to overcome resistance in biologically aggressive subtypes, WEE1 inhibition represents a compelling avenue for future therapeutic intensification.

5.4 Revisiting systemic therapy: Beyond cisplatin

Combination strategies involving cisplatin with lapatinib or tislelizumab have shown promise in p16-negative OPSCC. Lapatinib added to chemoradiation improved progression-free survival in this subgroup, while neoadjuvant tislelizumab plus chemotherapy demonstrated high pathological response rates. These approaches warrant further exploration to enhance outcomes in treatment-resistant, biologically aggressive disease [36, 37].

5.5 Radiation modulation and functional imaging

Dose de-escalation is not applicable in p16-negative OPSCC; instead, emphasis lies on optimizing local control. Functional imaging, such as hypoxia PET (FMISO PET) and diffusion-weighted MRI, can assist in adaptive radiotherapy, allowing dose escalation to resistant subvolumes without increasing toxicity. Emerging techniques such as dose painting modulating dose based on biological imaging are under evaluation and may help tailor radiation delivery in biologically aggressive tumors [38, 39].

5.6 Intensified chemoradiation for HPV-negative OPSCC

The DAHANCA 28 trial evaluated the feasibility of hyperfractionated accelerated radiotherapy (76 Gy/56 fractions) with weekly cisplatin and nimorazole in p16-negative head and neck cancers, including OPSCC. The regimen showed promising 3-year locoregional control and overall survival with manageable late toxicity but notable acute side effects. This study supports treatment intensification in biologically aggressive, HPV-negative disease and highlights the potential of hypoxia modification. It forms a basis for future trials focusing on biologically guided, adaptive, and patient-selective approaches to improve outcomes in this high-risk group [40].

5.7 Flash radiotherapy in p16-negative OPSCC: Emerging concept

Flash radiotherapy (FLASH-RT) is a novel technique that delivers radiation at ultra-high-dose rates (≥40 Gy/s) within milliseconds. Preclinical research suggests this approach can significantly reduce damage to normal tissues while maintaining effective tumor control—a phenomenon referred to as the "FLASH effect." In p16-negative OPSCC, where conventional treatment intensification is often constrained by toxicity, FLASH-RT offers the potential for safer dose escalation or hypofractionation. This could be particularly beneficial in overcoming resistance linked to tobacco-associated genomic alterations. Though still under investigation for head and neck cancers, FLASH-RT holds promise for enhancing the therapeutic ratio in this challenging setting [41].

5.8 Managing long-term toxicity and functional outcomes

Aggressive chemoradiation leads to a high burden of long-term morbidity, including feeding tube dependence, aspiration pneumonia, and fibrosis. Innovative

DOI: http://dx.doi.org/10.5772/intechopen.1012226

approaches in proton therapy and adaptive IMRT are being explored to minimize toxicity while maintaining control rates [42]. Structured supportive care pathways including swallowing therapy and early nutritional intervention will be integral components of future protocols for p16-negative disease.

Author details

Trinanjan Basu*, Rohith R. Menon, Jay P. Sahu and Ghazala K. Roshan
Department of Radiation Oncology, HCG Cancer Centre, Mumbai, India

*Address all correspondence to: trinanjan.doctor@gmail.com

References

[1] Elrefaey S, Massaro MA, Chiocca S, Chiesa F, Ansarin M. HPV in oropharyngeal cancer: The basics to know in clinical practice. Acta Otorhinolaryngologica Italica. 2014;**34**(5):299-309

[2] Machczynski P, Majchrzak E, Niewinski P, Marchlewska J, Golusinski W. A review of the 8th edition of the AJCC staging system for oropharyngeal cancer according to HPV status. European Archives of Oto-Rhino-Laryngology. 2020;**277**(9):2407-2412

[3] Sinha DN, Palipudi KM, Gupta PC, Singhal S, Ramasundarahettige C, Jha P. Smokeless tobacco use: A meta-analysis of risk and attributable mortality estimates for India. Indian Journal of Cancer. 2014;**51**(Suppl. 1):S73-S77

[4] Rischin D, Young RJ, Fisher R, Fox SB, Le QT, Peters LJ, et al. Prognostic significance of p16INK4A and human papillomavirus in patients with oropharyngeal cancer treated on the phase III trial TAX 324. Journal of Clinical Oncology. 2010;**28**(27):4142-4148

[5] Langendijk JA, Doornaert P, Verdonck-de Leeuw IM, Leemans CR, Aaronson NK, Slotman BJ. Impact of late treatment-related toxicity on quality of life among patients with head and neck cancer treated with radiotherapy. Journal of Clinical Oncology. 2008;**26**(22):3770-3776. DOI: 10.1200/JCO.2007.14.6647

[6] Mehanna H, Robinson M, Hartley A, et al. Radiotherapy plus cisplatin or cetuximab in low-risk HPV-positive oropharyngeal cancer (De-ESCALaTE HPV): An open-label randomised controlled phase 3 trial. Lancet. 2019;**393**(10166):51-60. DOI: 10.1016/S0140-6736(18)32752-1

[7] Maulik S, Roy P, Mallick I, Prasath S, Arun B, Chatterjee S. Definitive chemoradiation for oropharyngeal squamous carcinomas: Outcomes with intensity modulated radiation therapy using simultaneous integrated boost, in a majorly p16 negative cohort. Head and Neck. 2023;**45**(5):1156-1161. DOI: 10.1002/hed.27328

[8] Sarkar S, Ghosh A, Saha P, et al. Prevalence and prognostic significance of p16 and HPV in oropharyngeal squamous cell carcinoma: An Indian tertiary cancer center experience. Head & Neck. 2022;**44**(6):1246-1255. DOI: 10.1002/hed.27033

[9] Nguyen-Tan PF, Zhang Q, Ang KK, Weber RS, Rosenthal DI, Soulieres D, et al. Randomized phase III trial to test accelerated versus standard fractionation in combination with cisplatin for head and neck carcinomas: RTOG 0129. Journal of Clinical Oncology. 2014;**32**(27):2940-2950

[10] Ang KK, Zhang Q, Rosenthal DI, Nguyen-Tan PF, Sherman EJ, Weber RS, et al. Randomized phase III trial of concurrent accelerated radiation plus cisplatin with or without cetuximab for stage III to IV head and neck carcinoma: RTOG 0522. Journal of Clinical Oncology. 2014;**32**(27):2940-2950

[11] Pignon JP, le Maître A, Maillard E, Bourhis J, MACH-NC Collaborative Group. Meta-analysis of chemotherapy in head and neck cancer (MACH-NC): An update on 93 randomised trials and 17,346 patients. Radiotherapy and Oncology. 2009;**92**(1):4-14. DOI: 10.1016/j.radonc.2009.04.014

[12] Ang KK, Harris J, Wheeler R, Weber R, Rosenthal DI, Nguyen-Tân PF, et al. Human papillomavirus and survival of patients with oropharyngeal cancer. The New England Journal of Medicine. 2010;**363**(1):24-35

[13] Slaughter DP, Southwick HW, Smejkal W. Field cancerization in oral stratified squamous epithelium; clinical implications of multicentric origin. Cancer. 1953;**6**(5):963-968

[14] Leemans CR, Snijders PJF, Brakenhoff RH. The molecular landscape of head and neck cancer. Nature Reviews. Cancer. 2018;**18**(5):269-282. DOI: 10.1038/nrc.2018.11

[15] Ward MJ, Thirdborough SM, Mellows T, Riley C, Harris S, Suchak K, et al. Tumour-infiltrating lymphocytes predict for outcome in HPV-positive oropharyngeal cancer. British Journal of Cancer. 2014;**110**(2):489-500

[16] Beitler JJ, Zhang Q, Fu KK, et al. Final results of local-regional control and late toxicity of RTOG 9003: A randomized trial of altered fractionation radiation for locally advanced head and neck cancer. International Journal of Radiation Oncology, Biology, Physics. 2014;**89**(1):13-20

[17] Fu KK, Pajak TF, Trotti A, et al. A radiation therapy oncology group (RTOG) phase III randomized study to compare hyperfractionation and two variants of accelerated fractionation to standard fractionation radiotherapy for head and neck squamous cell carcinomas: First report of RTOG 9003. International Journal of Radiation Oncology, Biology, Physics. 2000;**48**(1):7-16. DOI: 10.1016/s0360-3016(00)00663-5

[18] Adelstein DJ, Li Y, Adams GL, et al. An intergroup phase III comparison of standard radiation therapy and two schedules of concurrent chemoradiotherapy in patients with unresectable squamous cell head and neck cancer. Journal of Clinical Oncology. 2003;**21**(1):92-98. DOI: 10.1200/JCO.2003.01.008

[19] Overgaard J, Hansen HS, Specht L, et al. Five compared with six fractions per week of conventional radiotherapy of squamous-cell carcinoma of head and neck: DAHANCA 6 and 7 randomised controlled trial: [published correction appears in Lancet. 2003 Nov 8;362(9395):1588]. Lancet. 2003;**362**(9388):933-940. DOI: 10.1016/s0140-6736(03)14361-9

[20] Denis F, Garaud P, Bardet E, et al. Final results of the 94-01 French head and neck oncology and radiotherapy group randomized trial comparing radiotherapy alone with concomitant radiochemotherapy in advanced-stage oropharynx carcinoma. Journal of Clinical Oncology. 2004;**22**(1):69-76. DOI: 10.1200/JCO.2004.08.021

[21] Bernier J, Cooper JS, Pajak TF, et al. Defining risk levels in locally advanced head and neck cancers: A comparative analysis of concurrent postoperative radiation plus chemotherapy trials of the EORTC (#22931) and RTOG (# 9501). Head & Neck. 2005;**27**(10):843-850. DOI: 10.1002/hed.20279

[22] Bourhis J, Overgaard J, Audry H, et al. Hyperfractionated or accelerated radiotherapy in head and neck cancer: A meta-analysis. Lancet. 2006;**368**(9538):843-854. DOI: 10.1016/S0140-6736(06)69121-6

[23] Lorch JH, Goloubeva O, Haddad RI, et al. Induction chemotherapy with cisplatin and fluorouracil alone or in combination with docetaxel in locally advanced squamous-cell cancer of the head and neck: Long-term results of the

TAX 324 randomised phase 3 trial. The Lancet Oncology. 2011;**12**(2):153-159. DOI: 10.1016/S1470-2045(10)70279-5

[24] Cooper JS, Zhang Q, Pajak TF, et al. Long-term follow-up of the RTOG 9501/intergroup phase III trial: Postoperative concurrent radiation therapy and chemotherapy in high-risk squamous cell carcinoma of the head and neck. International Journal of Radiation Oncology, Biology, Physics. 2012;**84**(5):1198-1205. DOI: 10.1016/j.ijrobp.2012.05.008

[25] Bourhis J, Sire C, Graff P, et al. Concomitant chemoradiotherapy versus acceleration of radiotherapy with or without concomitant chemotherapy in locally advanced head and neck carcinoma (GORTEC 99-02): An open-label phase 3 randomised trial. The Lancet Oncology. 2012;**13**(2):145-153. DOI: 10.1016/S1470-2045(11)70346-1

[26] Haddad R, O'Neill A, Rabinowits G, et al. Induction chemotherapy followed by concurrent chemoradiotherapy (sequential chemoradiotherapy) versus concurrent chemoradiotherapy alone in locally advanced head and neck cancer (PARADIGM): A randomised phase 3 trial. The Lancet Oncology. 2013;**14**(3):257-264. DOI: 10.1016/S1470-2045(13)70011-1

[27] Cohen EE, Karrison TG, Kocherginsky M, et al. Phase III randomized trial of induction chemotherapy in patients with N2 or N3 locally advanced head and neck cancer. Journal of Clinical Oncology. 2014;**32**(25):2735-2743. DOI: 10.1200/JCO.2013.54.6309

[28] Nichols AC, Theurer J, Prisman E, et al. Radiotherapy versus transoral robotic surgery and neck dissection for oropharyngeal squamous cell carcinoma (ORATOR): An open-label, phase 2, randomised trial. The Lancet Oncology. 2019;**20**(10):1349-1359. DOI: 10.1016/S1470-2045(19)30410-3 [published correction appears in Lancet Oncol. 2019 Dec;20(12):e663. doi: 10.1016/S1470-2045(19)30725-9]

[29] Machiels JP, Tao Y, Licitra L, et al. Pembrolizumab plus concurrent chemoradiotherapy versus placebo plus concurrent chemoradiotherapy in patients with locally advanced squamous cell carcinoma of the head and neck (KEYNOTE-412): A randomised, double-blind, phase 3 trial. The Lancet Oncology. 2024;**25**(5):572-587. DOI: 10.1016/S1470-2045(24)00100-1

[30] Lee NY, Ferris RL, Psyrri A, et al. Avelumab plus standard-of-care chemoradiotherapy versus chemoradiotherapy alone in patients with locally advanced squamous cell carcinoma of the head and neck: A randomised, double-blind, placebo-controlled, multicentre, phase 3 trial. The Lancet Oncology. 2021;**22**(4):450-462. DOI: 10.1016/S1470-2045(20)30737-3

[31] Patil VM, Noronha V, Joshi A, et al. A randomized phase 3 trial comparing nimotuzumab plus cisplatin chemoradiotherapy versus cisplatin chemoradiotherapy alone in locally advanced head and neck cancer. Cancer. 2019;**125**(18):3184-3197. DOI: 10.1002/cncr.32179

[32] Al-Mamgani A, van Rooij P, Verduijn GM, Mehilal R, Kerrebijn JD, Levendag PC. The impact of treatment modality and radiation technique on outcomes and toxicity of patients with locally advanced oropharyngeal cancer. The Laryngoscope. 2013;**123**(2):386-393. DOI: 10.1002/lary.23699

[33] Mirghani H, Amen F, Moreau F, Lacroix L, Marguet S, Urban T, et al. Human papilloma virus testing in

oropharyngeal squamous cell carcinoma: What is the issue? Journal of Clinical Medicine. 2019;**8**(5):622

[34] Jensen GL, Sun A, Birlea S, et al. Improved local control in p16-negative oropharyngeal cancers with hypermethylated MGMT. Radiotherapy and Oncology. 2021;**157**:234-240

[35] Kong A, Good J, Kirkham A, et al. Phase I trial of WEE1 inhibition with chemotherapy and radiotherapy as adjuvant treatment, and a window of opportunity trial with cisplatin in patients with head and neck cancer: The WISTERIA trial protocol. BMJ Open. 2020;**10**:e033009. DOI: 10.1136/bmjopen-2019-033009

[36] Kondo N, Tsukuda M, Ishiguro Y, Kimura M, Fujita K, Sakakibara A, et al. Antitumor effects of lapatinib (GW572016), a dual inhibitor of EGFR and HER-2, in combination with cisplatin or paclitaxel on head and neck squamous cell carcinoma. Oncology Reports. 2010;**23**:957-963

[37] Zhu J, Huang Y, Fang W, Wang F, Zhou T, Pan H, et al. Real-world study of neoadjuvant tislelizumab combined with chemotherapy in resectable locally advanced head and neck squamous cell carcinoma. Frontiers in Oncology. 2023;**13**:1160301. DOI: 10.3389/fonc.2023.1160301

[38] Giraud P, Le Rest CC, Espié M, Hatt M, Leboulleux S, Lasnon C, et al. Dose painting in radiotherapy for head and neck squamous cell carcinoma: Value of repeated functional imaging with ^{18}F-FDG PET, ^{18}F-fluoromisonidazole PET, diffusion-weighted MRI, and dynamic contrast-enhanced MRI. Journal of Nuclear Medicine. 2009;**50**(7):1020-1027

[39] van Elmpt W, De Ruysscher D, Lambin P. Biological PET-guided adaptive radiotherapy for dose escalation in head and neck cancer: A systematic review. Radiotherapy and Oncology. 2018;**129**(3):461-470

[40] Saksø M, Jensen K, Andersen M, Hansen CR, Eriksen JG, Overgaard J. DAHANCA 28: A phase I/II feasibility study of hyperfractionated, accelerated radiotherapy with concomitant cisplatin and nimorazole (HART-CN) for patients with locally advanced, HPV/p16-negative squamous cell carcinoma of the oropharynx, hypopharynx, larynx and oral cavity. Radiotherapy and Oncology. Jul 2020;**148**:65-72. DOI: 10.1016/j.radonc.2020.03.025. Epub 2020 Mar 28. PMID: 32335364

[41] Radiotherapy and Oncology, Favaudon V, Caplier L, Monceau V, Pouzoulet F, Sayarath M, et al. Ultrahigh dose-rate FLASH irradiation increases the differential response between normal and tumor tissue in mice. Science Translational Medicine. 2014;**6**(245):245ra93. DOI: 10.1126/scitranslmed.3008973

[42] Blanchard P, Gunn GB, Lin A, et al. Proton therapy for head and neck cancers. Seminars in Radiation Oncology. 2018;**28**(1):53-63

Chapter 4

Mediastinal Tracheostomy

Mihai-Dumitru Tudosie, Simona-Andreea Rujan, Bianca-Petra Taher, Gloria-Simona Bertesteanu, Alexandra Maria Marin, Raluca Grigore and Serban Vifor Gabriel Bertesteanu

Abstract

This chapter presents the case of a HPV-positive squamous-cell carcinoma of the larynx that underwent total laryngectomy with a tumoural recurrence after one year. The case is presented from admission in our clinic, the step-by-step salvage surgery and post-operative care. The pathology required a complex surgical technique involving mediastinal tracheostomy and double-flap reconstruction of the neck structures. The focus of the present study is on the technique used in mediastinal recalibration of the tracheal stoma.

Keywords: mediastinal tracheostomy, laryngeal cancer, head and neck surgery, flap reconstruction, tracheostomy

1. Introduction

Laryngeal cancer is one of the most frequent head and neck malignancies present in the general population, about 10.000 new cases being diagnosed each year. Stomal recurrence is a very serious complication after total laryngectomy, a meta-analysis reviewing cases for over 30 years shows that the most important risk factors are the tumour sub-site, the T stage before surgery, and positive resection margins after surgery [1]. Moreover, most often the recurrence presents in the first-year post-operative, but cases have been cited with tumoural recurrence at more than 3 years after surgery. Other risk factors that have been shown to affect the prognosis of stomal recurrence are previous tracheostomy, tumoural invasion of the thyroid gland, tracheal extension of the tumour, and other type of surgery upon the larynx (partial laryngectomies before the total laryngectomy) [2–6].

Anterior mediastinal tracheostomy is a surgical technique that involves removal of the manubrium and the reconfiguration of the tracheal stoma on the upper part of the thorax, instead of the base of the neck. It is a technique reserved for the cases in which the tumoural invasion involves the trachea and the cervical oesophagus, and it usually refers to the surgical treatment of stomal recurrence after total laryngectomy. It is a very challenging procedure, involving dissection along important blood vessels, such as the brachiocephalic trunk (innominate artery) and the common carotid arteries, a good control over reconstruction techniques, and a good cooperation with the anaesthetist, due to the apnoea steps involved [7–18].

2. Material and method

Biological constants, blood tests, and clinical progress were taken from the patient's observation sheet. All photographs were taken using a Samsung S20 smartphone. Consent of the patient regarding the photographic documentation and its use in this article was properly assured. Furthermore, a comprehensive study of the literature was involved in order to analyse the indications, contraindications, and opportunity of treatment in patients requiring this particular procedure.

3. Results: Surgical techniques

A 57-year-old patient, male, former smoker (~40pack-years, quit smoking for 5 years), chronic ethanol usage, post-total laryngectomy, presents for an induration of the region surrounding the tracheostomy, complaining of pain in the area and purulent discharge, dysphagia, and mild dyspnoea. History shows a histopathological result of HPV-positive squamous-cell carcinoma.

Clinical and endoscopic examination of the patient reveals status post-total laryngectomy, important salivary stasis in the oropharynx, and a tumoral growth around the tracheostomy, spreading towards the sternal insertion of the sternocleidomastoid (SCM) muscles bilaterally. Furthermore, stricture surrounding the tracheostomy was noted (**Figure 1**).

A CT-scan of head, neck, and thorax was performed in order to assess the local invasion and possible metastatic sites. Results revealed a tumoural process centred around the tracheostomy, invading the remaining hypo-pharynx and part of the cervical oesophagus circumferentially, the remaining SCM bilaterally, with extension in the superior mediastinum. After careful consideration, a discussion with the patient informing him about the risks associated with surgery, post-operative care

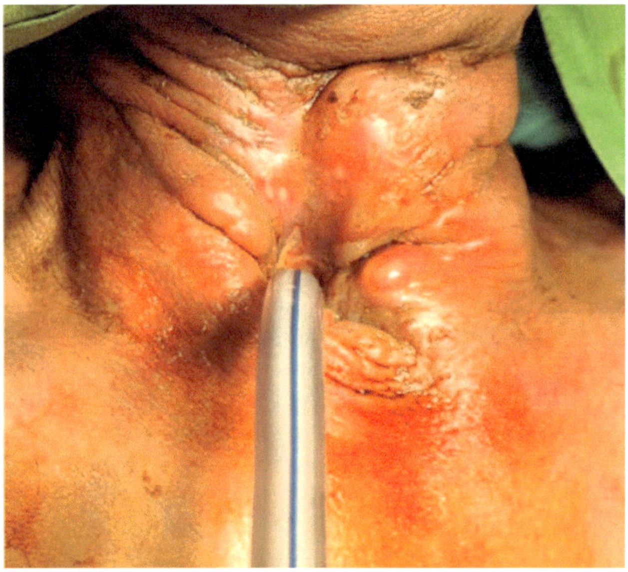

Figure 1.
Preoperative aspect.

and obtaining consent, the case was analysed in a tumour-board that agreed with the salvage surgery.

Preoperative preparation involved antibioprophylaxis with wide-spectrum antibiotics, thromboprophylaxis, stress-ulcer prophylaxis, and balance of physiological constants.

Surgery began with an incision circumventing the tumour, allowing wide access and evaluation the extension of said tumour (**Figures 2** and **3**).

After initial evaluation of tumour extension bilateral lateral neck dissection was performed in order to expose the main neurovascular bundle of the neck (internal jugular vein, common carotid artery, and vagus nerve) (**Figures 4** and **5**).

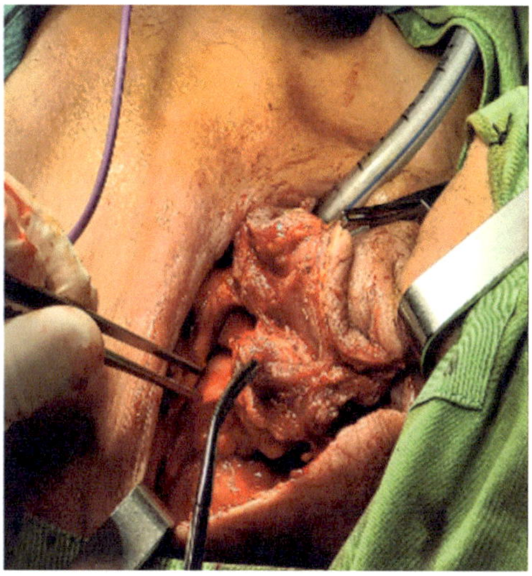

Figure 2.
Incision and evaluation of tumoural extension.

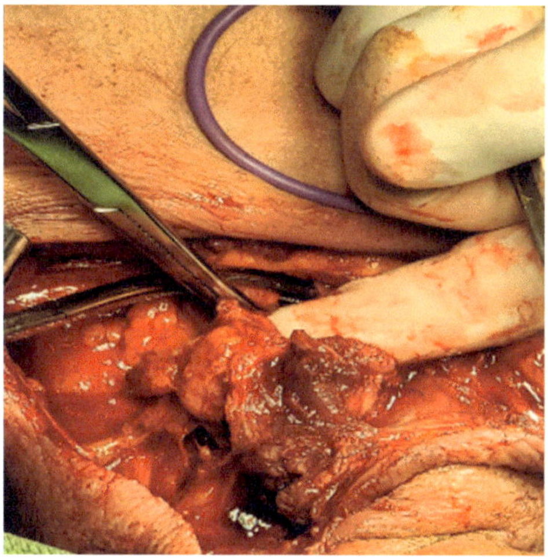

Figure 3.
Evaluation of tumoural extension (close-up).

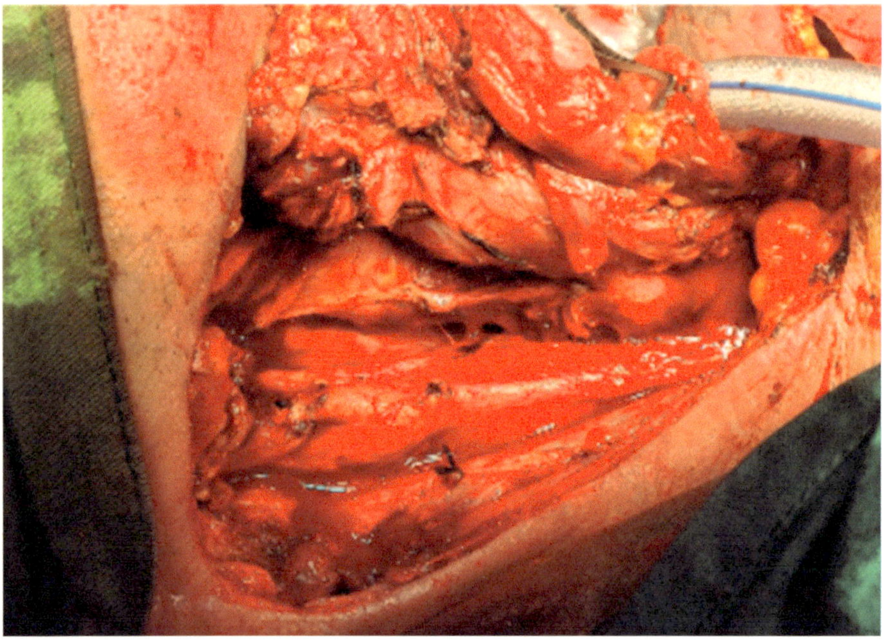

Figure 4.
Right lateral neck dissection.

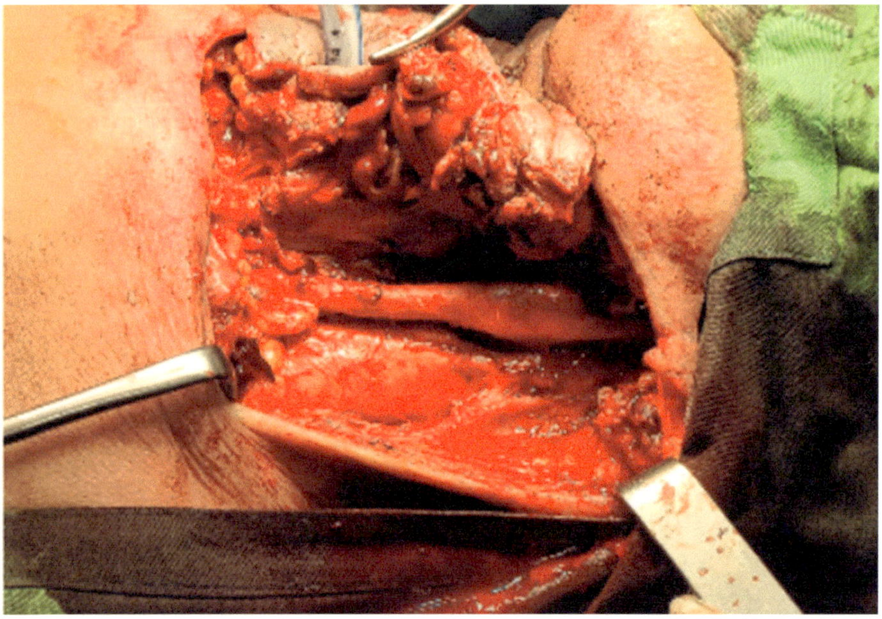

Figure 5.
Left lateral neck dissection. Forceps are placed on the inferior end of the resected internal jugular vein. Ligation of the external carotid artery was performed above the superior thyroid artery.

While performing the lateral neck dissection invasion of the left internal jugular vein was noticed, therefore the internal jugular vein was resected en-bloc with the tumour. Moreover, invasion of the inferior branches of the left external carotid artery required ligation and resection of the left external carotid artery.

After ensuring the integrity of the major vessels of the neck, superior and inferior dissection was performed. Superior dissection followed the tumour alongside its superior margin (ensuring a safe resection margin). Inferior, the tumour was invading 4 tracheal cartilages, and therefore, extending the dissection into the superior mediastinum was necessary (**Figures 6** and 7). After the tracheal resection, we were able to evaluate the posterior aspect of the tumour and the posterior extension (**Figure 8**).

The intraoperative view confirmed that the CT findings, the entire hypo-pharynx, and the superior part of the cervical oesophagus were involved.

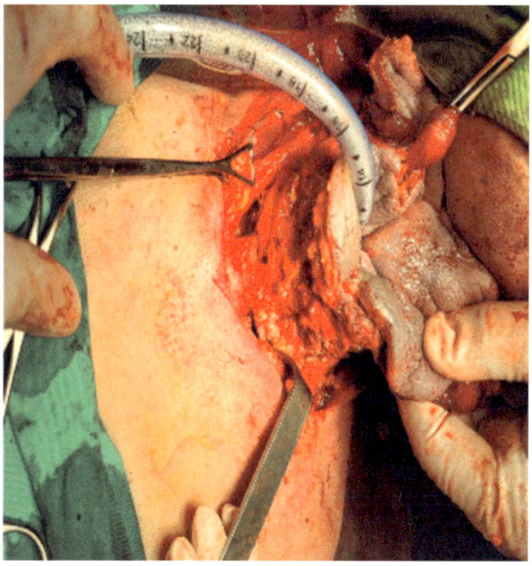

Figure 6.
Inferior dissection into the superior mediastinum.

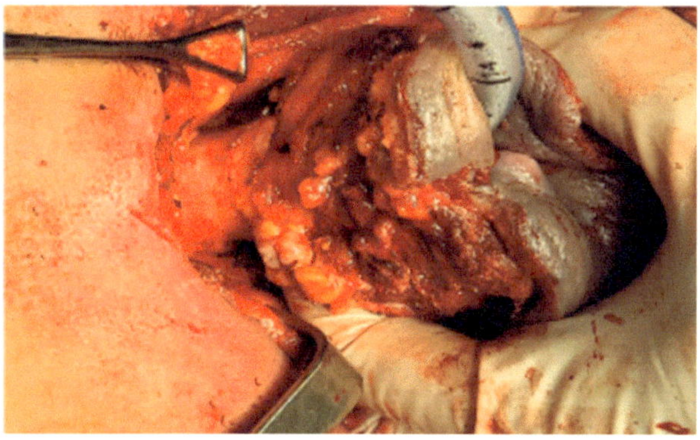

Figure 7.
Inferior dissection into the superior mediastinum, exposing the trachea until finding healthy tissue.

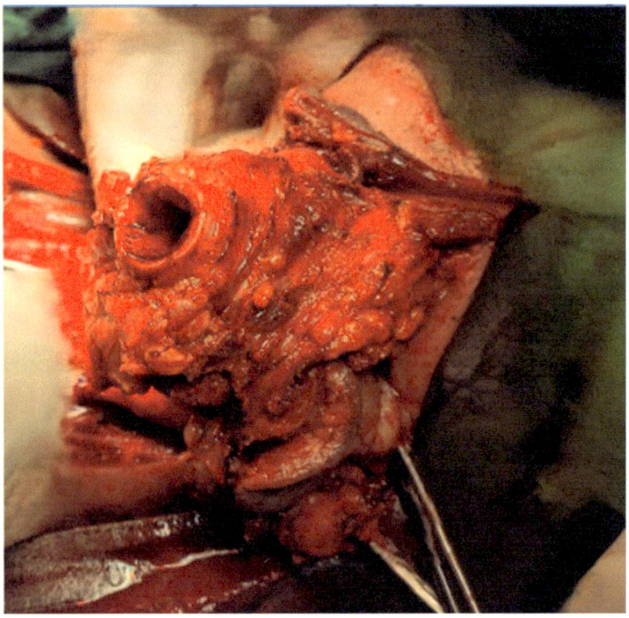

Figure 8.
Evaluation of the posterior aspect and removal of the tumour en-bloc with the hypo-pharynx and cervical oesophagus.

Resection of the tumour left an enormous defect involving the entire anterior cervical region, a short trachea that could not be lifted in order to make a proper cervical tracheostoma, and a circular defect of the upper digestive tract from the base of the tongue almost to the thoracic part of the oesophagus (**Figures 9-11**).

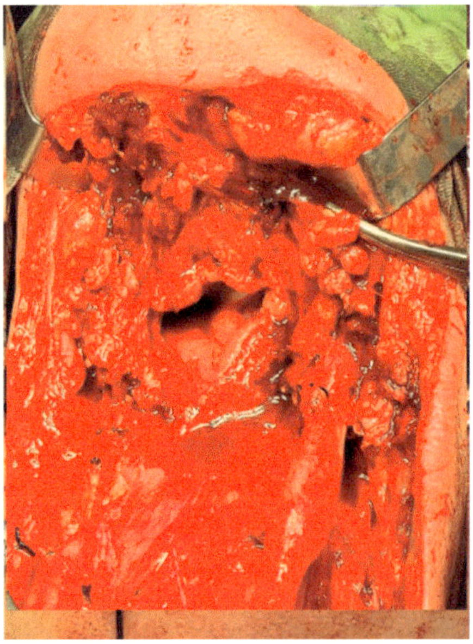

Figure 9.
Digestive tract defect, superior side.

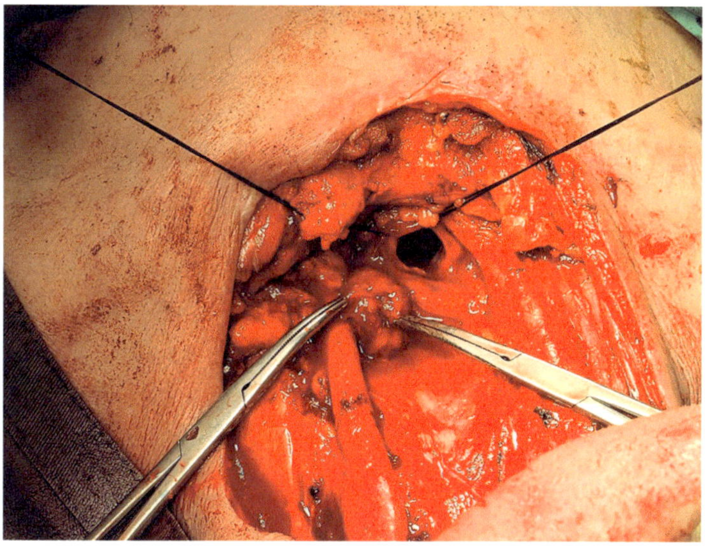

Figure 10.
Defect after tumoural resection, inferior side. Oesophagus held by forceps. Trachea anchored by wire.

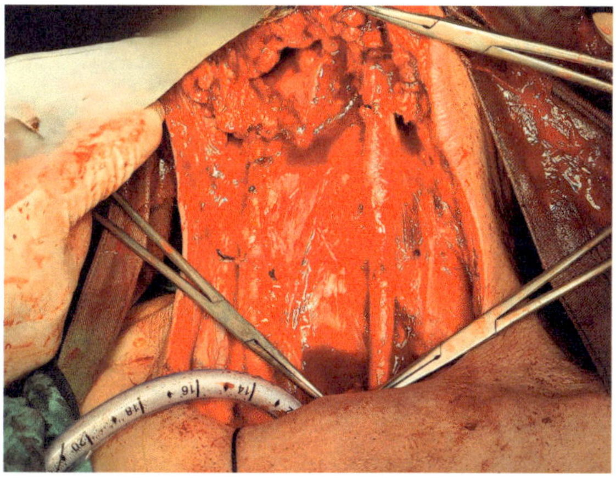

Figure 11.
Overview of the surgical defect.

This posed the very challenging task of reconstruction, in order to assure a continuous digestive tract, a patent tracheostomy without traction on the trachea and closing a gigantic skin defect. Therefore, we decided on performing the following:

1. Mediastinal tracheostomy

2. Reforming of the digestive continuity using a pectoral flap folded upon itself

3. Closure of the skin defect with a pectoral flap prelevated from the contralateral pectoral region.

3.1 Mediastinal tracheostomy

A midline incision along the upper chest was executed, along with the dissection of the soft tissue until reaching the manubrium. Afterwards, a superior sternotomy was performed, in order to expose the thoracic trachea, alongside the brachiocephalic trunk. In order to prevent erosion of the trunk, a transposition between the trachea and the brachiocephalic trunk is mandatory, pulling the end of the trachea under the vessel. In this case, the vessel is in contact with the muscular and not the cartilaginous part of the trachea (**Figures 12** and **13**). The final step in creating a mediastinal tracheostoma is to anchor the opening of the trachea to the skin, as shown in **Figure 14**. Reconstruction of the remaining defect will be shown in the next steps.

3.2 Reforming of the digestive continuity

This particular step of the surgery remains the most challenging, due to the lack of prosthetic materials required to reconstruct the esopharyngeal wall. As an alternative, we used a piece of an intubation tube as a mentor on which we placed a pectoralis major flap. The pectoral flap is the ENT surgeon's "work-horse" as it provides more than enough tissue in order to create a neo-pharynx. We prelevated a regional pectoralis major flap from the left side, as shown in **Figures 15-18**.

Once put in place, we used a piece of intubation tube as a guide and mentor in order to reconstruct the digestive tract. This step represented a challenge due to the inexistence of proper prosthetic devices that could allow a more physiological development of the flap in order to become part of the digestive tract. The mentor was anchored with surgical wire through the nose for easy removal afterwards. Sutures of both ends of the digestive tract defect and sutures of the flap onto itself in order to create a "tube" were performed (**Figures 19-22**).

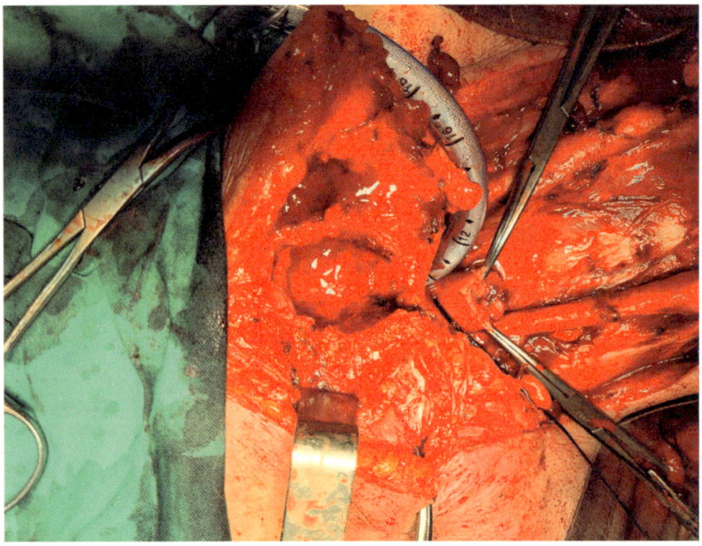

Figure 12.
Removal of the sternal manubrium.

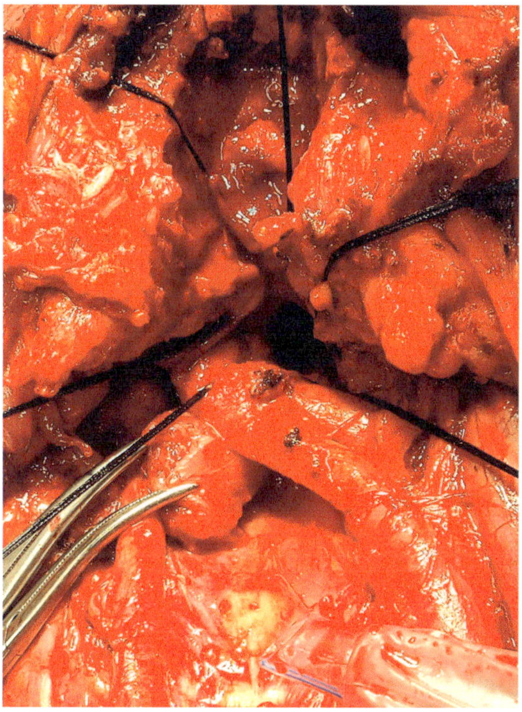

Figure 13.
Approximation of the trachea in order to pass under the innominate artery.

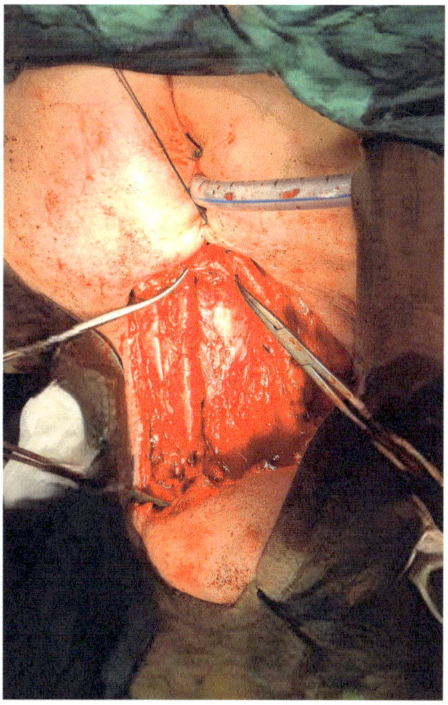

Figure 14.
Closure of the mediastinum and anchoring the trachea.

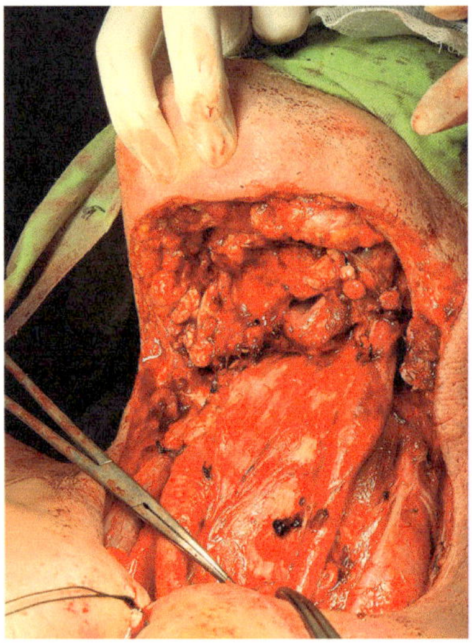

Figure 15.
Magnitude of the anterior cervical defect.

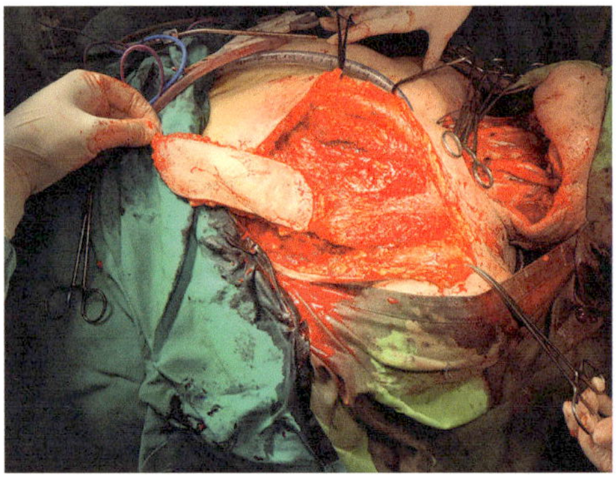

Figure 16.
Prelevation of the pectoralis major flap on the left side.

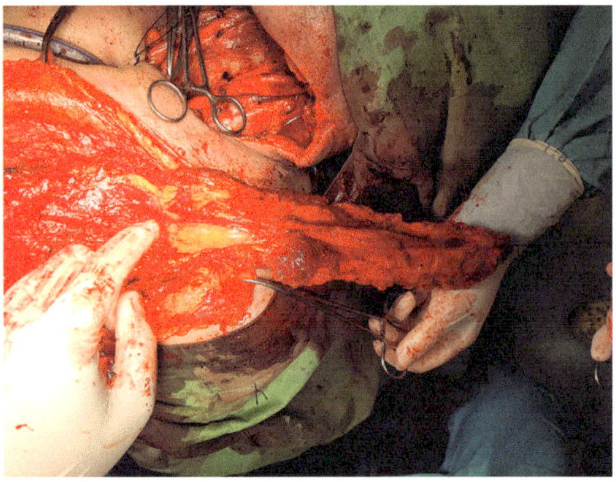

Figure 17.
Identification of the pediculum.

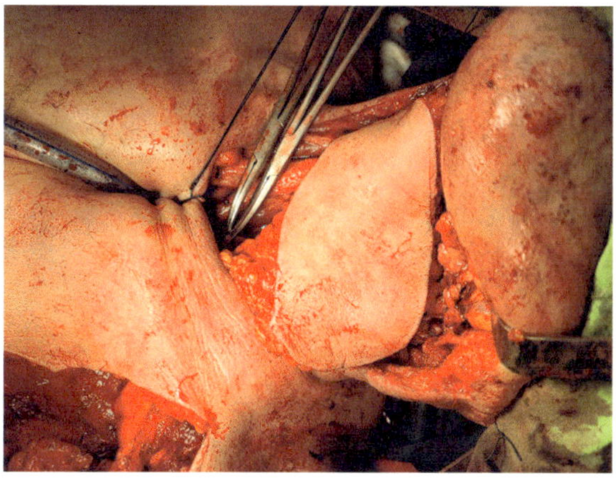

Figure 18.
Approximation of the flap's position.

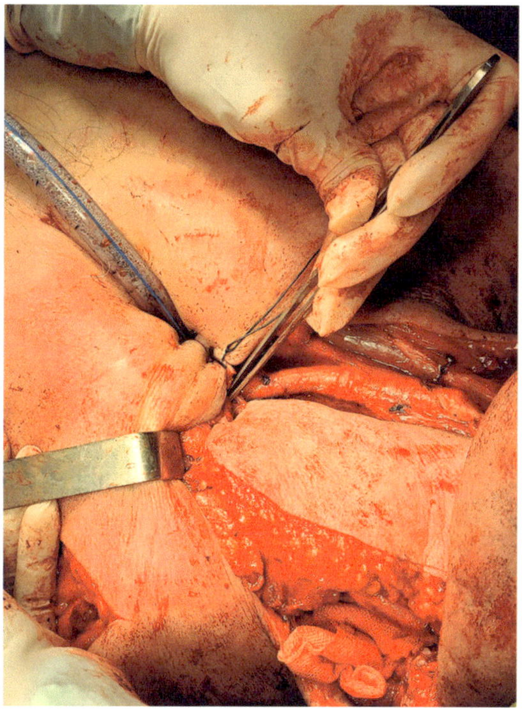

Figure 19.
Sutured flap to the ends of the defect.

3.3 Closure of the skin defect with a pectoral flap from the contralateral pectoral region

After resolving the placement of the new tracheostoma and reconstruction of the digestive tract, the cervical skin defect still remained an issue. Due to the poor quality of the tissues remaining in the cervical region after previous surgery and radiotherapy, we decided that the most feasible solution will be another regional flap,

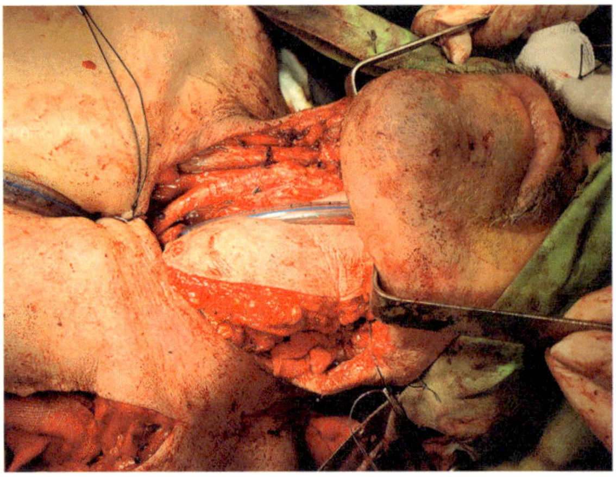

Figure 20.
Placement of the mentor in order to perform the tubulisation.

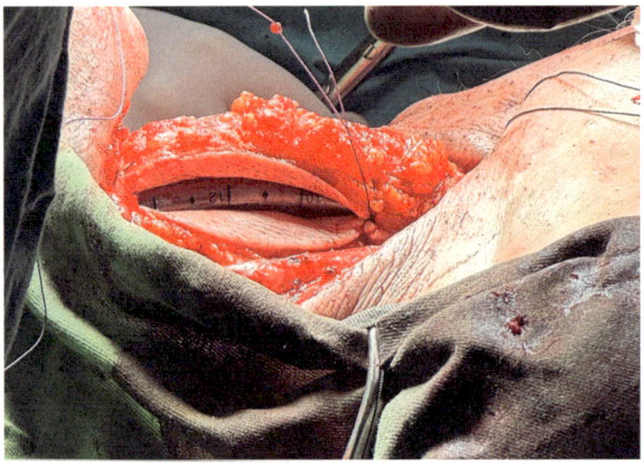

Figure 21.
Closure of the pectoral flap.

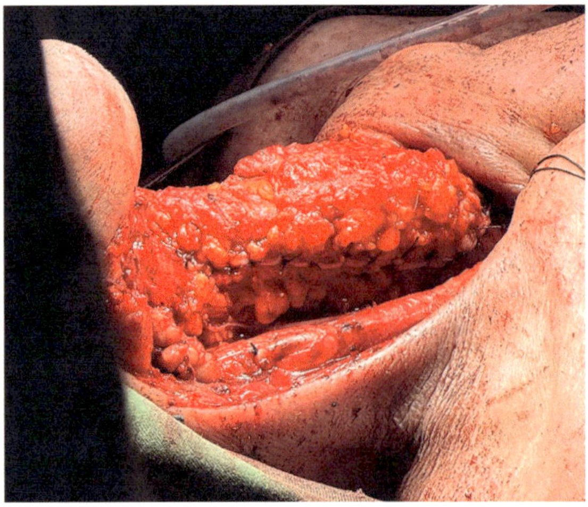

Figure 22.
Aspect after complete closure.

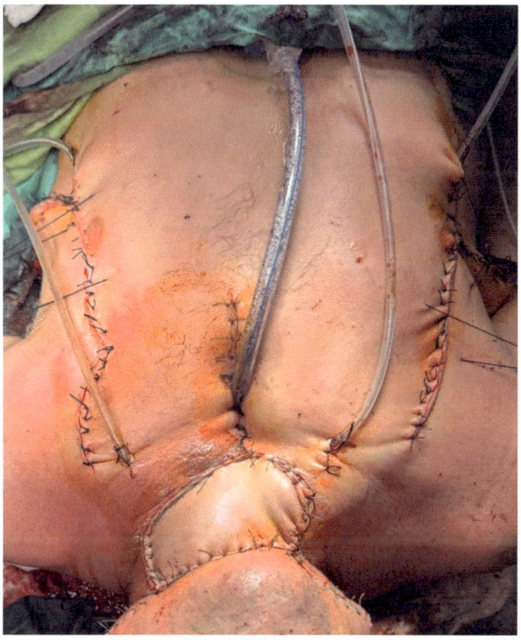

Figure 23.
Aspect at the end of surgery.

from the contralateral site. Closure of the defect was performed in multi-layer technique, ensuring no tension and no pressure on the flaps (**Figure 23**). As an additional method of protection against tears in the sutures, we applied thoracic-menton wires to prevent hyperextension of the head.

Post-operative care remains a critical stage in the evolution of the patient, our primary concern being the very high risk of fistulas, necrosis of the flaps or important bleeding due to extensive dissection around major blood vessels. Unfortunately, after a few days, due to poor tissue vascularisation and difficult cooperation with the patient (not complying with our recommendation to avoid swallowing of saliva, no head extension, etc.) he developed a fistula. We decided on a conservative approach of the fistula, assuring a dry wound that will allow secondary granulation and closure.

4. Conclusions

1. Tumoural recurrence of the tracheostoma is a rare pathology that implies a lot of resources in its management, and it is usually considered inoperable.

2. Mediastinal tracheostomy is considered salvage surgery after all other possibilities have been used, such as radiotherapy and chemotherapy.

3. Stomal recurrence usually involves the invasion of the hypo-pharynx and/or the cervical oesophagus, and therefore, a reconstructive technique should always be known by the surgical team.

4. Always bring the opening of the tracheostoma under the brachiocephalic trunk in order to prevent the erosion of the blood vessel and secondary massive haemorrhage.

5. Consider approaching the case in multidisciplinary team (general surgeon and plastic surgeon) and prepare a good preoperative plan, taking into account any possible incidents that may occur.

6. Mediastinal tracheostomy provides local disease control and can restore airway continuity in selected patients, but it is rarely curative due to the advanced tumour stage at presentation.

7. Surgical morbidity is high, and complications such as infection, vascular erosion, and flap failure are not uncommon. Reported survival remains limited, reflecting the palliative or salvage nature of the intervention.

8. Outcomes depend heavily on the experience of the surgical team and the availability of reconstructive options; centres with established multidisciplinary collaboration achieve better results.

9. Careful patient selection is paramount. Candidates should be evaluated not only for technical operability but also for performance status, prior treatments, and expected quality of life.

10. In modern practice, mediastinal tracheostomy is best regarded as a salvage but function-preserving procedure, aiming to alleviate symptoms, reduce the risk of life-threatening airway compromise, and, in select cases, prolong survival.

Acknowledgements

This study was funded by "Carol Davila" University of Medicine and Pharmacy, Bucharest. The authors express their gratitude to the University for providing the financial support.

Notes/thanks/other declarations

We would like to express our profound gratitude to Professor Serban Vifor Gabriel Bertesteanu for his generous provision of research materials and his invaluable guidance throughout the preparation of this work. We also wish to acknowledge the members of his research team, whose dedicated efforts in gathering information and materials provided essential support to the successful completion of this paper.

Author details

Mihai-Dumitru Tudosie[1,2*], Simona-Andreea Rujan[1,2], Bianca-Petra Taher[1,2], Gloria-Simona Bertesteanu[1,3], Alexandra Maria Marin[1,2], Raluca Grigore[1,2] and Serban Vifor Gabriel Bertesteanu[1,2]

1 "Carol Davila" University of Medicine and Pharmacy, Bucharest, Romania

2 ENT Department of "Coltea" Clinical Hospital, Bucharest, Romania

3 ENT Department of Central Military Hospital, Bucharest, Romania

*Address all correspondence to: mihai-dumitru.tudosie@drd.umfcd.ro

References

[1] Liang J, Zhu X, Zeng W, Yu T, Fang F, Zhao Y. Which risk factors are associated with stomal recurrence after total laryngectomy for laryngeal cancer? A meta-analysis of the last 30 years. Brazilian Journal of Otorhinolaryngology. 2020;**86**(4):502-512. DOI: 10.1016/j.bjorl.2020.03.002. Epub 2020 Apr 11

[2] Kowalski LP, Rinaldo A, Robbins KT, Pellitteri PK, Shaha AR, Weber RS, et al. Stomal recurrence: Pathophysiology, treatment and prevention. Acta Oto-Laryngologica. 2003;*123*(3):421-432. DOI: 10.1080/00016480310000683a

[3] Conti M, Benhamed L, Mortuaire G, Chevalier D, Pinçon C, Wurtz A. Indications and results of anterior mediastinal tracheostomy for malignancies. The Annals of Thoracic Surgery. 2010;**89**(5):1588-1595. DOI: 10.1016/j.athoracsur.2010.01.044

[4] Bagheri R, Rahim MB, Majidi M, et al. Anterior mediastinal tracheostomy for malignancy: Analysis of 12 cases. Asian Cardiovascular & Thoracic Annals. 2013;**21**(2):187-192. DOI: 10.1177/0218492312456849

[5] Berthet J-P, Garrel R, Dubruc E, et al. Anterior mediastinal tracheostomy as salvage operation. The Annals of Thoracic Surgery. 2014;**98**(3):972-978. DOI: 10.1016/j.athoracsur.2014.05.050

[6] Martinod E, Guillaume JY, Radu DM, Despreaux G. A more conservative technique for anterior mediastinal tracheostomy after sub-total resection of the trachea. Interactive Cardiovascular and Thoracic Surgery. 2011;**12**(5):672-674. DOI: 10.1510/icvts.2010.257170

[7] Gomes MN et al. Mediastinal tracheostomy. The Annals of Thoracic Surgery. 1987;**43**(5):539-543

[8] Berthet J-P et al. Anterior mediastinal tracheostomy as salvage operation. The Annals of Thoracic Surgery. 2014;**98**(3):1026-1033

[9] Yamamoto Y et al. Simple palliative mediastinal tracheostomy. The Annals of Thoracic Surgery. 2013;**95**(6):2185-2187

[10] Chew KY, Kok YO, Ong WL, Tan BK. Coverage of anterior mediastinal tracheostomy with bipedicled anterolateral thigh flap. JPRAS Open. 2021;**28**:4-9. DOI: 10.1016/j.jpra.2021.01.007

[11] Liu PH, Hung CJ, Tseng YL, Lee YC. Chimeric anterolateral thigh flap for one-stage reconstruction after cervical exenteration with anterior mediastinal tracheostomy. Plastic and Reconstructive Surgery. Global Open. 2022;**10**(7):e4444. DOI: 10.1097/GOX.0000000000004444

[12] Chan YW, Yu Chow VL, Lun Liu LH, Ignace WW. Manubrial resection and anterior mediastinal tracheostomy: Friend or foe? Laryngoscope. 2011;**121**(7):1441-1445. DOI: 10.1002/lary.21852. Epub 2011 May 18

[13] Kuwabara Y, Sato A, Mitani M, Shinoda N, Hattori K, Suzuki T, et al. Use of omentum for mediastinal tracheostomy after total laryngoesophagectomy. The Annals of Thoracic Surgery. 2001;**71**(2):409-413. DOI: 10.1016/s0003-4975(00)02228-1

[14] Fujita H, Kakegawa T, Yamana H, Shirouzu G, Minami T. Mediastinal tracheostomy using a pectoralis major myocutaneous flap after resection of carcinoma of the esophagus involving the proximal part of the trachea. Surgery, Gynecology & Obstetrics. 1990;**171**(5):403-408

[15] Chen C, Liu S, Zhao G, et al. Application of low anterior mediastinal tracheostomy for cervicothoracic esophageal cancer with long-segment tracheal involvement: A case report. Annals of Esophagus. 2021;**5**:5. DOI: 10.21037/aoe-20-94

[16] Wurtz A, De Wolf J. Anterior mediastinal tracheostomy: Past, present, and future. Thoracic Surgery Clinics. 2018;**28**(3):277-284. DOI: 10.1016/j.thorsurg.2018.03.002

[17] Hartert M, Hillebrand C, Kass E, et al. Anterior mediastinal tracheostomy as Mission: Impossible. Journal of Thoracic Disease. 2021;**13**(12):7189-7192. DOI: 10.21037/jtd-21-1617

[18] Mayer N, Sandu K, Chung JH, et al. Surgical access to the mediastinum—All roads lead to Rome. Journal of Thoracic Disease. 2024;**16**(4):1131-1149. DOI: 10.21037/jtd-24-134

Chapter 5

Role of Metronomic Chemotherapy in Advanced Oral Cancer

Rohan Thomas Mathew and Anu Babu

Abstract

Oral squamous cell carcinoma (OSCC) is a significant global health burden, with a disproportionately high incidence and mortality in low- and middle-income countries, often due to the advanced-stage diagnosis. Conventional palliative chemotherapy is frequently inaccessible due to cost and toxicity. Metronomic chemotherapy involves the regular administration of low, less-toxic doses of chemotherapeutic drugs over prolonged periods, with no extended drug-free breaks. Unlike maximum-tolerated dose chemotherapy scheduling, which directly targets tumour cells, metronomic chemotherapy primarily acts on the vascular endothelial cells in the tumour stroma. Metronomic chemotherapy regimens—involving methotrexate, celecoxib, and erlotinib—offer comparable or superior survival outcomes to conventional palliative chemotherapy in advanced, recurrent, refractory, or metastatic OSCC. It is also associated with significantly reduced toxicity, fewer hospitalisations, and improved quality of life. Oral administration and cost-effectiveness make it particularly suited for resource-constrained settings, reducing financial and time toxicity for patients. While challenges regarding patient compliance and monitoring persist, metronomic chemotherapy is presently the standard of care for palliative patients. Metronomic therapy has also been used for neoadjuvant therapy, bridge therapy, and even as maintenance therapy. It has also been used with immunotherapy, highlighting the versatility of metronomic chemotherapy in advanced oral cancer.

Keywords: oral cancer, OSCC, recurrent OSCC, metronomic chemotherapy, palliative care, methotrexate, celecoxib

1. Introduction

Head and neck cancers, particularly oral squamous cell carcinoma (OSCC), are a significant public health problem. Globally, OSCC is the sixth most common cancer. The incidence of OSCC in South Asia and Southeast Asia is significantly higher. It is one of the most common cancers in India. There are about 77,000 new cases and 52,000 deaths due to oral cancer, one of the highest incidences in the world, with an increasing trend in India [1]. There is also a disparity in incidence and outcomes of OSCC between the developed and developing countries. The lower socioeconomic status can contribute to the increased incidence, along with the other common risk factors, such as areca nut, smokeless tobacco, smoking tobacco and alcohol, with smoking and alcohol often acting synergistically. There is also a significant increase in the incidence of oral cancer in individuals under the age of 45 [2]. This shows a worrying trend where the younger population is getting affected by oral cancer, possibly due to the early onset of tobacco usage. Consequently, the Disability-Adjusted Life Year (DALY), mortality rate, and the resulting loss of productivity due to oral cancer have increased significantly over the past two decades. The rate of annual incidence is also growing more so in South Asia and Southeast Asia [3].

There have been numerous advances in the management of oral cancer. Extensive surgical resections are possible due to improvements in microvascular reconstruction, anaesthesia, and better understanding of the tumour biology. Side effects arising from radiotherapy are also decreasing with advanced machines, which can deliver the planned dose to the target volume, sparing the skin and other adjacent structures. The role of chemotherapy is limited in oral cancer. Neoadjuvant chemotherapy has resulted in organ preservation but does not translate to better overall survival. Recent trials, such as the Keynote 689 and EXTREME trials, have highlighted the role of targeted therapy and immunotherapy in HNSCC. However, these advances have not changed much of the overall survival of patients. It is about 60–70% in the high-income countries, whereas it is between 40 and 50% in the low- and low-middle-income countries [2]. One of the reasons for poorer overall outcomes is the advanced stage at diagnosis. Close to 70% of the patients have locoregional disease at the time of diagnosis [4]. Present treatment guidelines dictate that these patients receive multimodality treatment; however, due to the advanced nature of the disease, these patients have early recurrence or residual disease, which are not amenable to salvage. Conventional management deems them incurable and would provide palliative chemotherapy or palliative care alone, which involves managing the symptoms of the patient, without changing the course of the disease. Chemotherapy regimens, which are recommended by the National Comprehensive Cancer Network (NCCN) for palliation in HNSCC, are not widely used in low- and low-middle-income countries due to their cost. Metronomic chemotherapy has been shown to be better suited for these patients with limited side effects and similar overall outcomes [5].

Metronomic chemotherapy is the regular administration of low, less-toxic doses of chemotherapeutic drugs for prolonged periods of time with no extended drug-free breaks [6]. A metronome is a musical device which produces regular audible clicks that represent a regular pulse, like the regular administration of drugs. The metronomic doses are usually 1/10th to 1/3rd of the maximum tolerated dose (MTD). This differs from the conventional philosophy, which aims to kill as many tumour cells as possible by giving the maximum dose of chemotherapy that the patient can tolerate. Metronomic chemotherapy works by a different mechanism, which requires a

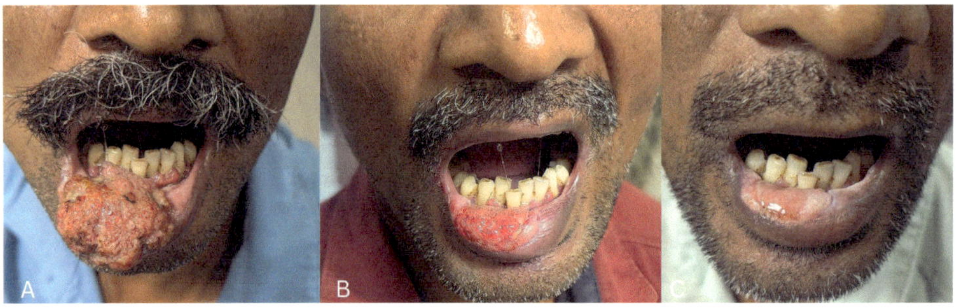

Figure 1.
A: Tumour at presentation. B: Regression of tumour after the first dose. C: Regression after the second dose.

constant low blood level of the drug. The low dose also ensured that the patients had limited or no associated toxicities [7].

With the preclinical evidence of antiangiogenic action of metronomic chemotherapy, it was first tried in refractory cases and in palliative care. It was tried in breast, colorectal, ovarian and other solid organ malignancies with variable results [8–10].

Currently, metronomic chemotherapy plays a significant role in palliative care. This is exceptionally effective in HNSCC and particularly in OSCC. The role in cases with curative intent is still being studied. Along with palliative care, the authors are also using metronomic chemotherapy for patients who are waiting for the definitive treatment, often with a significant reduction in tumour size (**Figure 1**).

2. History

Conventional cytotoxic chemotherapy is based on cell line studies and mathematical models deriving the survival curves for cancer-cell kill. The aim is to completely eradicate the cancer cells. These multi-drug regimens are used to kill as many tumour cells as possible. Few researchers have identified the potential therapeutic implications of neo-angiogenesis, which is one of the hallmarks of cancer. It was postulated by Folkan in 1971 that the growth of solid organ cancers is always accompanied by neovascularisation caused by tumour angiogenesis. He suggested that the therapeutic interventions targeting angiogenesis can lead to novel treatment strategies [11]. Following this, multiple novel molecules were identified as potential drugs, which can target various angiogenic pathways with variable results.

In the late 1990s, experimental studies have proven that low and frequent doses are more effective in anti-angiogenesis than a single large bolus followed by long rest periods [12].

Low and frequent dose of conventional cytotoxic drugs was initially described as an anti-angiogenic scheduling of chemotherapy. Based on the work by Browder et al. [13] and Klement et al. [14], it was Douglas Hanahan and team who termed it metronomic chemotherapy [15].

This principle was then tested preclinically with different drugs and cell lines [16, 17].

The idea was then translated clinically by repurposing the cytotoxic drugs and using them in palliative patients. It was tried in various solid organ malignancies, such as breast, colorectal, and ovarian cancers with good results, slowly making towards regular oncological practice [8–10].

In oral cancer, it was first tried in patients with advanced disease who had a waiting period of more than 3 weeks. A retrospective analysis of the data was done, and they found that the majority of the patients responded to the metronomic chemotherapy, and the overall outcomes were better with these patients compared to the patients who did not receive it [18].

Following this, the same group did numerous other studies to study the drugs, dosage, and the efficacy of metronomic chemotherapy in oral cancer. Presently, it is standard of care for palliative care.

3. Mechanism of action

Metronomic chemotherapy is the administration of less toxic, low doses of chemotherapy at regular intervals for prolonged periods of time with no extended drug-free breaks. The conventional cytotoxic chemotherapy aims to kill as many cancer cells as possible by the administration of the maximum tolerable dose (MTD). This is achieved by damaging the DNA and the DNA repair mechanisms. Metronomic chemotherapy acts on angiogenesis and immune modulation.

Numerous studies have identified the various pathways involved in angiogenesis and how to develop molecules to target these. This also highlights the importance of the tumour-host interface and the role of the microenvironment in initiation, invasion, and progression of the tumour. Malignant cells are adept at inducing changes in the local microenvironment to ensure their survival. This includes abnormal stimulation of the immune and inflammatory cell functions and inducing angiogenesis. A better understanding of the cellular and molecular pathways and growth factors involved has resulted in identifying several targets, which can potentially be used for inhibiting angiogenesis, such as vascular endothelial growth factor (VEGF), angioproteins, and receptor tyrosine kinase expressed by the endothelial cells of newly formed vessels. This has led to the development of drugs that block the receptors for VEGF or the angioproteins [12, 14].

Extensive research has also identified various molecules which have antiangiogenic properties, and some of the conventional cytotoxic drugs can target the tumour endothelial cells in low and frequent doses. Early in vitro and in vivo studies have shown these results in a significant reduction of the tumour volume [13, 14].

Metronomic chemotherapy primarily acts on the tumour endothelial cells. These cells, unlike the endothelium of mature blood vessels, proliferate rapidly and are susceptible to cytotoxic agents. However, long intervals between the cycles, such as the case of conventional chemotherapy, will allow the survival and regrowth of a fraction of these cells, resulting in persistent neovascularisation of the tumour [12, 15].

Hypoxia factor (HIF-1α) and VEGF are pro-angiogenetic factors, which are stimulated in a hypoxic microenvironment. In some studies, metronomic chemotherapy has decreased the circulating HIF-1α levels. The endothelial progenitor cells, which also play a significant role in the neovascularisation, are also targeted by metronomic chemotherapy. It also induces antiangiogenic protein thrombospondin-1, which inhibits HIF-1α, which in turn decreases circulating VEGF levels [19].

The second aspect of metronomic chemotherapy is by modulation of the immune system of the host. It selectively depletes the regulatory T cell, which plays an important role in tumour immune tolerance. This will lead to the restoration of the natural killer cells and T cell function, enhancing the antitumor immune response. Metronomic chemotherapy also induces antigen-presenting dendritic cell maturation, which increases its tumorigenic antigen presentation, causing immunogenic cancer death [20].

Non-cytotoxic doses of doxorubicin, methotrexate, and mitomycin C improved the ability of dendritic cells to present tumour antigens to T-cells in vitro. This resulted in the upregulation of multiple molecules on the dendritic cell surface, such as CD80, CD86, CD40, and MHC Class II. Along with these, increased production of IL-1β, IL-6, and IL-12 was also identified in low concentrations of vinblastine and vinorelbine. Several cytotoxic drugs, such as methotrexate, at low concentrations could increase the ability of dendritic cells to induce T-cell proliferation through enhancing these cells' maturation and antigen presentation [19].

There are also other mechanisms which are proposed for the effect of metronomic chemotherapy. Cancer stem cells (CSCs) are tumour-initiating cells that are resistant to conventional cytotoxic chemotherapy. In certain preclinical models, it was identified that metronomic chemotherapy with antiangiogenic drugs reduced the CSC population [21].

Inducing tumour dormancy is also considered to be a potential mechanism of action of metronomic chemotherapy. It is postulated to work by inducing angiogenic dormancy, cellular dormancy (tumour cells in G0–G1 arrest), and immunosurveillance (preventing residual tumour cells from expanding) [7].

4. The difference between conventional cytotoxic chemotherapy and metronomic chemotherapy

Cytotoxic, conventional antiproliferative agents are still part of the treatment for advanced head and neck cancers. The presently accepted model for these agents is multidrug regimens designed to kill as many tumour cells as possible by administering at the maximum tolerated dose (MTD). The limiting factor in these regimens is the tolerability of the patient. For this, a high dose of chemotherapy is given in a day or a few days, followed by 3–4 weeks of rest, to allow the normal cells to recover, particularly the bone marrow. Bone marrow suppression can result in serious complications.

Solid organ tumours are notorious for multiple genetic abnormalities and for a heterogeneous subpopulation of cells with different cell kinetics, angiogenic, invasive, and metastatic properties. This will lead to a variable response to the chemotherapeutic regimen, even in the same patient. Our recent understanding of the tumour microenvironment, the stroma, also does not fit into the conventional cytotoxic chemotherapy. Targeting just the cancer cells is not always enough to control the long-term outcomes, particularly the risk of developing distant metastasis [12].

Metronomic chemotherapy targets the surrounding stromal tissue, particularly the endothelial cells, which have a high proliferative index. Lower doses, administered

	Conventional cytotoxic chemotherapy	Metronomic chemotherapy
Primary target	Tumour cells directly	Stromal tissue, especially endothelial cells
Dose strategy	Maximum tolerated dose (MTD)	Low doses (1/3 to 1/10 of MTD)
Administration schedule	High dose in a day followed by 3–4 weeks of rest, fixed number of cycles	Continuous, frequent low-dose administration
Model basis	Log-dose survival curve (from leukaemia cell lines in mice)	Anti-angiogenic action of drugs
Main limiting factor	Patient tolerability (bone marrow suppression, toxicity)	Disease progression or intolerable side effects
Toxicity and side effects	High; serious complications possible (e.g., bone marrow suppression)	Much lower; better tolerance
Route of administration	Often intravenous, hospital-based	Mostly oral; fewer hospital visits
Tumour response	Variable due to genetic heterogeneity and microenvironment	Targets angiogenesis and stromal support rather than tumour heterogeneity
Treatment duration	Fixed cycles	Continuous until progression or side effects
role in care	Major role in curative treatment; some role in palliative	Mostly studied in palliative care; potential expansion in future

Table 1.
Comparison between conventional chemotherapy and metronomic chemotherapy.

frequently, cytotoxic drugs predominantly target these rapidly proliferating endothelial cells, sparing other cells. This results in considerably lower side effects, leading to improved tolerance. The low dose and mostly by oral routes mean that the patients need not visit the hospital frequently.

Conventional cytotoxic chemotherapy is explained by the log-dose survival curve model. This model was developed on mice cell lines with leukaemia and has been used for chemotherapy dose calculations. Whereas, the metronomic chemotherapy dose is determined by the anti-angiogenic action of these drugs. The dosages are usually one-third to one-tenth of the MTDs. The exact doses are based on experimental data and the clinical acumen of the oncologists. While conventional chemotherapy is always given for fixed cycles, metronomic chemotherapy is given continuously until there is disease progression or intolerable side effects. The key differences are highlighted in **Table 1**.

The role of metronomic chemotherapy beyond palliative care is still being studied. Conventional cytotoxic chemotherapy still has a major role to play in curative treatment and some role in palliative chemotherapy as well. The roles may diminish in future with a better understanding of the tumour biology, introduction of targeted therapy, and immunotherapy.

5. Role of metronomic chemotherapy in advanced oral cancer

Patients with oral cancers often present at advanced stages, which require multimodality treatment with surgery, radiotherapy, and occasionally chemotherapy. The role of neoadjuvant chemotherapy (NACT) is well studied in head and neck squamous cell carcinoma (HNSCC). In loco-regionally advanced cases, NACT is given in selected cases, which is followed by definitive chemoradiotherapy or surgery. Although some of the patients will have a good response after NACT, it has not significantly translated to improvement in survival benefits. Multi-agent regimens, which are the standard of care, lead to increased complications, such as stomatitis, diarrhoea, neutropenia, and febrile neutropenia. This has led to an increased number of patients not completing the planned definitive radiotherapy or surgery. Moreover, most of the patients from low-middle-income countries (LMIC) are from a lower socioeconomic background and are poorly nourished to begin with. Many of these countries have a high incidence of oral cancer. Due to various reasons, more than 60% of the patients report to the hospital at an advanced stage with locoregional spread. This has led to an increased burden on the public health infrastructure, which treats cancer patients, where the patients may have to wait up to 30 days before the commencement of treatment [4].

Metronomic chemotherapy was first tried in OSCC patients during this time, between diagnosis and definitive treatment. A retrospective study was conducted in a tertiary cancer centre in India to document and analyse the effect of metronomic chemotherapy in pretreatment patients of OSCC. Notably, 32 patients were enrolled in the study. The regimen was oral methotrexate 15 mg/m^2 weekly once and oral celecoxib 200 mg twice daily, until the previous day of surgery. The role of methotrexate in HNSCC is well documented, and in an earlier study, it was identified that 15 mg/m^2 saturates the tumour dihydrofolate reductase. Hence, any further escalation would have limited value [22].

Cyclo-oxygenase-2 (COX-2) is upregulated in inflammation, neovascularisation and in neoplasms. Celecoxib is a COX-2 inhibitor, which will result in reduced angiogenesis and downregulation of pro-angiogenic factors. Along with this, celecoxib also plays a role in the suppression of cell proliferation and the induction of apoptosis [23].

The drugs were restarted a week after surgery. Patients underwent adjuvant treatment based on the final histopathology as per the standard guidelines. During the adjuvant therapy, methotrexate was withheld and started again 4 weeks after the completion of the treatment with the intention to continue for 18 months. The regimen was well tolerated, and most of the patients were compliant. The patients were able to take the drugs at their homes, and they did not have to visit a hospital during the time due to any complications. The data, which was analysed, found that this regimen has a response rate of 75%. Further analysis using the Kaplan-Meier method estimated that the group which received metronomic chemotherapy had a 14.9% improvement in the 2-year disease-free survival (DFS) [18].

Based on this data, a phase 2 prospective randomised controlled trial was done by the same team in patients with recurrent, metastatic or locally advanced HNSCC who were eligible for palliative chemotherapy. There were 110 patients enrolled in this study. The investigators compared single-agent cisplatin on one arm, and in the other arm, patients received daily oral celecoxib 200 mg twice daily and oral methotrexate 15 mg/m^2 weekly. The results show an improvement in the progression-free survival with oral metronomic chemotherapy compared to intravenous cisplatin. There were fewer overall toxicities and adverse events in the metronomic arm. The patients also had fewer non-protocol hospital visits. This highlights the better tolerance for this arm. It is also more suited for home-based care, specifically in places where access to a tertiary cancer care is restricted by financial or geographical constraints. This also eases the resources in an already resource-constrained health infrastructure [24].

A phase 3 prospective randomised study was also done with 422 enrolled patients who had recurrence, relapse, or locally advanced cases, and who were planned for palliative chemotherapy. The patients were randomly assigned to the oral metronomic chemotherapy group and the intravenous cisplatin group. The drug dosage and scheduling were not changed. This study reiterated the prior findings that metronomic chemotherapy improves survival, higher quality of life, and reduced adverse effects [5].

Other combinations were also tried with some success. Methotrexate, along with cetuximab, was tried in recurrent or metastatic HNSCC. Cetuximab is a recombinant human/mouse chimeric monoclonal antibody which binds to EGFR and inhibits the receptor activation by competing with epidermal growth factor. EGFR is upregulated in the majority of head and neck cancers. The results showed cetuximab with methotrexate improved the outcomes without increased toxicity [25, 26].

Another recent trial compared triple metronomic chemotherapy comprising erlotinib, methotrexate, and celecoxib. While metronomic chemotherapy acts by anti-angiogenesis, erlotinib acts on multidrug transporters, such as ABCC2, ABCC3, and ABCG2, which expel methotrexate from cancer cells, which are linked to resistance and poor prognosis, thereby enhancing the action of the metronomic chemotherapy. In this phase 3 randomised controlled trial, triple OMCT is compared to chemotherapy of the physician's choice. The study enrolled 214 patients, and their outcomes were analysed. The study showed improvement in OS in the metronomic group. This is one of the few studies which showed improved OS in a palliative setting which does not use immunotherapy. The toxicities are also less than those of conventional chemotherapy. The control group also showed an improvement in quality-of-life measurements and reduced unplanned hospitalisations [27].

Another group of researchers from Taiwan studied the effect of metronomic chemotherapy when given as a maintenance therapy after the completion of the treatment with curative intent. They used Tegafur-uracil. It is a 4:1 molar mixture of uracil and tegafur. Tegafur is a pro-drug of fluorouracil, which gets converted into its active form by the cytochrome P-450 enzyme. Uracil is an inhibitor of the fluorouracil-degrading enzyme dihydropyrimidine dehydrogenase. This ensures a stable plasma concentration of 5-FU with low toxicity. It was given at a daily dose of 100–400 mg for 3–9 months. Although the study was done in HNSCC patients, majority of them were OSCC patients. The results show that patients who underwent the maintenance metronomic therapy with tegafur-uracil had better benefits for patients who took the drugs longer [28, 29].

There is adequate evidence presently to use metronomic chemotherapy in recurrent or metastatic or platinum-resistant cases. However, there is no consensus on its role in the neoadjuvant setting.

A study from Japan did a retrospective analysis to compare the use of S-1, an oral fluoropyrimidine anticancer agent, in metronomic doses as neoadjuvant therapy vs. upfront surgery. S-1 monotherapy was given to patients who could not be scheduled for surgery for various reasons. They found out that the patients who received S-1 had a significantly higher overall survival. It was more effective in patients with moderately differentiated or poorly differentiated cases than in well-differentiated cases [30].

Another study from a tertiary cancer centre administered the triple oral metronomic chemotherapy regimen comprising methotrexate, celecoxib, and erlotinib to patients as a neoadjuvant protocol during the waiting period for surgery, as a 'bridge therapy'. This ranged from 2 to 6 weeks, with most of the patients receiving for 4 weeks. They analysed the patients' final histopathology to understand the histomorphological changes and the tumour response after administering the triple metronomic chemotherapy. In a sample size of 50, 2 patients had a pathological complete response, 3 patients had no response, and the remaining 45 patients showed a partial response. In patients for whom there was no response, the disease progressed in two patients. However, there was some response in 95% of the patients [31].

This highlights the different aspects of metronomic chemotherapy in OSCC. It also highlights the variability of tumour biology. There is still no uniformity in the response, and to treat the patients optimally, close follow-up is essential, especially while giving it as a neoadjuvant protocol.

Low-dose immunotherapy has also been tried with the triple oral metronomic chemotherapy with good outcomes. Pembrolizumab and nivolumab are checkpoint inhibitors, which are being tried in platinum-refractory recurrent HNSCC [32]. Low-dose nivolumab (20 mg flat dose once every 3 weeks), along with oral methotrexate, celecoxib, and erlotinib, is compared with the same regimen without nivolumab. Patients continued to receive the therapy until the development of intolerable side effects or progression. The study showed significant improvement in outcomes with the addition of low-dose nivolumab, along with the triple oral metronomic chemotherapy, with no increase in adverse events [33].

In a recently conducted systematic review on the efficacy of oral metronomic chemotherapy in the management of head and neck cancers, there is strong evidence to support the use of metronomic chemotherapy in head and neck cancers, particularly oral cancers. Administration of metronomic chemotherapy resulted in higher survival and response rate in patients when compared to standard chemotherapy [34].

6. Advantages and disadvantages of metronomic chemotherapy in advanced oral cancer

The morbidity and mortality arising from oral cancer has led to a loss of productivity, increasing the economic burden on the patient and the caretaker. The cost of premature mortality due to oral cancer in India is $5.6 billion per annum. This is 0.18% of the combined gross domestic product (GDP) [35]. This also has a significant drain on the public health infrastructure, which predominantly manages these patients. These centres are few in number and are overwhelmed with the increasing incidence of oral cancer. Travelling to these centres is also an issue for the patients since they require an overnight journey to reach the centre.

More than the loss of productivity of the patient, there is also the loss of wages for the bystander who is accompanying the patient. Hence, it is essential that newer modalities of treatment are introduced so that the patient does not need to travel frequently. Metronomic chemotherapy has been adopted across India quickly for these reasons. They are cost-effective for the patients, who can take these medicines continuously without a significant drain on their savings. They are usually given for oral administration; hence the visit to the hospital is completely avoided, unless there are some complications. Lower doses usually do not result in serious adverse events which require hospitalisation. The lower side effects, reduced hospitalisation, and reduced travel will improve the quality of life for the patient and the family. The oncological outcomes of metronomic therapy are also comparable to palliative regimens of conventional chemotherapy, but without the side effects and hospitalisation. The palliative care patients in whom metronomic chemotherapy is administered have similar oncological outcomes, reduced financial toxicity, and reduced time toxicity.

Earlier, the patients who had recurrent, refractory and incurable disease were usually deemed palliative intent and were not given anti-cancer treatment. The patient's priority also would be to spend more time with the family and have fewer health issues. Metronomic chemotherapy has helped them live a reasonably symptom-free life with improved quality of life and reduced health issues and hospitalisations.

The major drawback of metronomic therapy is that it relies heavily on the compliance of the patients to take the right drugs and right time. It has been our experience that some patients forget to take the weekly tablets. The efficiency will be affected if the constant dose is not maintained. Another limitation is the lack of constant follow-up which would identify progression of disease. It could be an increase in size or formation of new lesions. In metronomic scheduling, patients are reviewed only once in 3 months. On one hand, this would help reduce the cost of travelling and the associated loss of productivity, but on the other hand, the patients are not being seen for 3 months. Disease progression, which requires change of drugs, is missed in this period. Metronomic therapy is not without any complications. Some patients do develop skin rashes, fatigue, oral mucositis, etc. The tolerance of the patients to these side effects is variable. While some patients tolerate the side effects well, some do not. They need to be individualised and titrated to get the best results. Methotrexate can also result in neutropenia rarely. The major advantages and disadvantages are shown in **Table 2**.

This is a dreaded complication and needs hospitalisation for the management. The patients who are on metronomic chemotherapy should check their blood count and renal function regularly. Impaired renal functions can also cause untoward complications. Patients should be advised to report back to a nearby hospital if any complication occurs.

Advantages	Disadvantages
Cost-effective for patients	Relies on patient compliance; missed doses reduce efficacy
Oral administration, reduces need for hospital visits	Infrequent follow-up may miss disease progression
Lower side effects compared to conventional/ palliative chemotherapy	Potential complications: skin rashes, fatigue, oral mucositis, neutropenia, and renal complications
Reduced need for hospitalisation, travel, and reduced time toxicity	Requires regular blood count and renal function checks
Improved quality of life and symptom control with reduced financial toxicity	Some patients experience poor tolerance to side effects; dosing must be individualised

Table 2.
Advantages and disadvantages of metronomic chemotherapy.

7. Conclusion

Metronomic scheduling of chemotherapy is a promising avenue in head and neck cancers, particularly oral cancer. Over the past few years, it has emerged as an important therapeutic strategy in the management of advanced oral cancers, particularly in a resource-constrained setup. While conventional chemotherapy continues to play a vital role in curative and a limited role in palliative settings, the evidence increasingly supports the use of metronomic chemotherapy, especially in recurrent, refractory, and metastatic diseases. Clinical studies and trials have demonstrated comparable or superior survival outcomes, improved tolerance, and reduced hospitalisation rates, supporting its position as a viable standard of care in palliative management and as a bridge in curative settings. However, challenges remain regarding patient compliance, regular monitoring, and individualisation of therapy, which are critical for optimising outcomes.

Going forward, with further refinement in drug combinations, better protocols for follow-up, and integration with newer modalities, such as targeted therapy and immunotherapy, metronomic chemotherapy is poised to assume a greater role in the future management of oral cancer. Its ability to extend survival, reduce suffering, and maintain dignity in patients who would otherwise have limited therapeutic options marks it as a significant advancement in oncological practice, particularly in the fight against oral cancer in high-burden regions.

Conflict of interest

The authors declare no conflict of interest.

Author details

Rohan Thomas Mathew[1*] and Anu Babu[2]

1 Head and Neck Division, Department of Surgical Oncology, Zulekha Yenepoya Institute of Oncology, Yenepoya Medical College and Hospital, Yenepoya (Deemed to be University), Mangalore, India

2 Department of Oral Medicine and Radiology, Yenepoya Dental College, Yenepoya (Deemed to be University), Mangalore, India

*Address all correspondence to: rohanthomas@gmail.com

References

[1] Akashanand ZQS, Jena D, Ballal S, Kumar S, Bhat M, et al. Burden of oral cancer and associated risk factors at national and state levels: A systematic analysis from the global burden of disease in India, 1990-2021. Oral Oncology. 2024;**159**:107063

[2] Sun R, Dou W, Liu W, Li J, Han X, Li S, et al. Global, regional, and national burden of oral cancer and its attributable risk factors from 1990 to 2019. Cancer Medicine. 2023;**12**(12):13811-13820

[3] Wang Y, Zhuo L, Yang S, Dong C, Hu X. The worldwide epidemiology of lip and oral cavity cancer attributable to smoking based on the global burden of disease study 2019. Journal of Public Health. 2025;**33**(5):1135-1144

[4] Babu A, Mathew RT, Shetty R. Pattern of oral cancer in India: An analysis of hospital based cancer registry data. Journal of Indian Academy of Oral Medicine and Radiology. 2023;**35**(4):497

[5] Patil V, Noronha V, Dhumal SB, Joshi A, Menon N, Bhattacharjee A, et al. Low-cost oral metronomic chemotherapy versus intravenous cisplatin in patients with recurrent, metastatic, inoperable head and neck carcinoma: An open-label, parallel-group, non-inferiority, randomised, phase 3 trial. The Lancet Global Health. 2020;**8**(9):e1213-e1222

[6] Bocci G, Kerbel RS. Pharmacokinetics of metronomic chemotherapy: A neglected but crucial aspect. Nature Reviews. Clinical Oncology. 2016;**13**(11):659-673

[7] De Felice F, Musio D, Tombolini V. Head and neck cancer: Metronomic chemotherapy. BMC Cancer. 2015;**15**(1):677

[8] Kamat AA, Kim TJ, Landen CN, Lu C, Han LY, Lin YG, et al. Metronomic chemotherapy enhances the efficacy of antivascular therapy in ovarian cancer. Cancer Research. 2007;**67**(1):281-288

[9] Kaur H, Budd GT. Metronomic therapy for breast cancer. Current Oncology Reports. 2004;**6**(1):49-52

[10] Fioravanti A, Canu B, Alì G, Orlandi P, Allegrini G, Di Desidero T, et al. Metronomic 5-fluorouracil, oxaliplatin and irinotecan in colorectal cancer. European Journal of Pharmacology. 2009;**619**(1-3):8-14

[11] Folkman J. Tumor angiogenesis: Therapeutic implications. The New England Journal of Medicine. 1971;**285**(21):1182-1186

[12] Gasparini G. Metronomic scheduling: The future of chemotherapy? The Lancet Oncology. 2001;**2**(12):733-740

[13] Browder T, Butterfield CE, Kräling BM, Shi B, Marshall B, O'Reilly MS, et al. Antiangiogenic scheduling of chemotherapy improves efficacy against experimental drug-resistant cancer. Cancer Research. 2000;**60**(7):1878-1886

[14] Klement G, Baruchel S, Rak J, Man S, Clark K, Hicklin DJ, et al. Continuous low-dose therapy with vinblastine and VEGF receptor-2 antibody induces sustained tumor regression without overt toxicity. The Journal of Clinical Investigation. 2000;**105**(8):R15-R24

[15] Hanahan D, Bergers G, Bergsland E. Less is more, regularly: Metronomic dosing of cytotoxic drugs can target tumor angiogenesis in mice. The Journal of Clinical Investigation. 2000;**105**(8):1045-1047

[16] Wang J, Lou P, Lesniewski R, Henkin J. Paclitaxel at ultra low concentrations inhibits angiogenesis without affecting cellular microtubule assembly. Anti-Cancer Drugs. 2003;**14**(1):13-19

[17] Pasquier E, Honore S, Pourroy B, Jordan MA, Lehmann M, Briand C, et al. Antiangiogenic concentrations of paclitaxel induce an increase in microtubule dynamics in endothelial cells but not in cancer cells. Cancer Research. 2005;**65**(6):2433-2440

[18] Pai PS, Vaidya AD, Prabhash K, Banavali SD. Oral metronomic scheduling of anticancer therapy-based treatment compared to existing standard of care in locally advanced oral squamous cell cancers: A matched-pair analysis. Indian Journal of Cancer. 2013;**50**(2):135

[19] Muraro E, Vinante L, Fratta E, Bearz A, Höfler D, Steffan A, et al. Metronomic chemotherapy: Anti-tumor pathways and combination with immune checkpoint inhibitors. Cancers. 2023;**15**(9):2471

[20] Simsek C, Esin E, Yalcin S. Metronomic chemotherapy: A systematic review of the literature and clinical experience. Journal of Oncology. 2019;**2019**:5483791

[21] Kareva I, Waxman DJ, Klement GL. Metronomic chemotherapy: An attractive alternative to maximum tolerated dose therapy that can activate anti-tumor immunity and minimize therapeutic resistance. Cancer Letters. 2015;**358**(2):100-106

[22] Schifeling DJ, George T, McGuirt F, Capizzi RL, Kamen BA. Methotrexate content in squamous cell carcinoma of the head and neck after low-dose methotrexate. Medical and Pediatric Oncology. 1994;**22**(2):88-90

[23] Bock JM, Menon SG, Sinclair LL, Bedford NS, Goswami PC, Domann FE, et al. Celecoxib toxicity is cell cycle phase specific. Cancer Research. 2007;**67**(8):3801-3808

[24] Patil VM, Noronha V, Joshi A, Muddu VK, Dhumal S, Bhosale B, et al. A prospective randomized phase II study comparing metronomic chemotherapy with chemotherapy (single agent cisplatin), in patients with metastatic, relapsed or inoperable squamous cell carcinoma of head and neck. Oral Oncology. 2015;**51**(3):279-286

[25] Ham JC, Van Meerten E, Fiets WE, Beerepoot LV, Jeurissen FJF, Slingerland M, et al. Methotrexate plus or minus cetuximab as first-line treatment in a recurrent or metastatic (R/M) squamous cell carcinoma population of the head and neck (SCCHN), unfit for cisplatin combination treatment, a phase Ib-randomized phase II study commence. Head and Neck. 2020;**42**(5):828-838

[26] Sukari A, Nagasaka M, Diab M, Al Sibai K, Atassi B, Elayoubi JA, et al. Cetuximab and methotrexate in recurrent or metastatic head and neck squamous cell carcinoma—A single institution analysis of 54 patients. Clinical Otolaryngology. 2019;**44**(4):639-643

[27] Kapoor A, Gupta A, Sansar B, Mishra BK, Gupta P, Singh A, et al. Triple oral metronomic chemotherapy versus chemotherapy of physician discretion after failure of platinum-based therapy in advanced head and neck cancer: A phase III randomized study (METRO-CHASE study). JCO Global Oncology. 2025;**11**:e2500032

[28] Hsieh MY, Chen G, Chang DC, Chien SY, Chen MK. The impact of

metronomic adjuvant chemotherapy in patients with advanced oral cancer. Annals of Surgical Oncology. 2018;**25**(7):2091-2097

[29] Yeh TJ, Chan LP, Tsai HT, Hsu CM, Cho SF, Pan MR, et al. The overall efficacy and outcomes of metronomic Tegafur-uracil chemotherapy on locally advanced head and neck squamous cell carcinoma: A real-world cohort experience. Biology. 2021;**10**(2):168

[30] Kina S, Miyamoto S, Kawabata-Iwakawa R, Kina-Tanada M, Ogawa M, Yokoo S. Higher overall survival rates of oral squamous cell carcinoma treated with metronomic neoadjuvant chemotherapy. American Journal of Cancer Research. 2024;**14**(3):1033-1051

[31] Aravind S, Jose J, Shenoy PK, Avaronnan M, Thavarool SB, Nayanar SK. The spectrum of histomorphological changes and pathological tumor response following preoperative oral metronomic chemotherapy in oral squamous cell carcinoma. South Asian Journal of Cancer. 2022;**11**(2):146-151

[32] Ferris RL, Blumenschein G, Fayette J, Guigay J, Colevas AD, Licitra L, et al. Nivolumab for recurrent squamous-cell carcinoma of the head and neck. The New England Journal of Medicine. 2016;**375**(19):1856-1867

[33] Patil VM, Noronha V, Menon N, Rai R, Bhattacharjee A, Singh A, et al. Low-dose immunotherapy in head and neck cancer: A randomized study. Journal of Clinical Oncology. 2023;**41**(2):222-232

[34] Segin Chandran AB, Pandiar D, Krishnan RP, Gopinath D. Efficacy of oral metronomic chemotherapy in the management of head and neck squamous cell carcinoma—A systematic review. Frontiers in Oral Health. 2025;**6**:1632316

[35] Singh A, Sullivan R, Bavaskar M, Shetty R, Joshi P, Nair S, et al. A prospective health economic evaluation to determine the productivity loss due to premature mortality from oral cancer in India. Head and Neck. 2024;**46**(6):1263-1269

Chapter 6

Stereotactic Body Radiotherapy in Head and Neck Malignancy

Shwetima Chaudhary, Abiramasundari V and Vishwadeep Mishra

Abstract

Stereotactic body radiotherapy (SBRT) is a very focused and on-target form of radiotherapy used for treatment in head and neck tumors. It delivers strong, targeted radiation doses to kill directly to the tumor, while protecting nearby healthy tissues. This approach is very helpful for patients with recurrent or advanced-stage cancers, where standard treatments may not be effective. Studies show SBRT can achieve good local control and survival rates, even in complex cases. Its accuracy makes it suitable for tumors in difficult-to-reach areas, offering new options for patients who were previously considered untreatable. However, careful planning is essential to account for tumor size, location, and nearby critical structures. SBRT is a crucial path forward in head and neck cancer tumor, for improving outcomes and maintaining the good quality of life for many patients.

Keywords: SBRT, head and neck cancers, local control, critical, accuracy

1. Introduction

Oncologists have had a bitter experience with recurrent, previously irradiated malignancy of the head and neck with palliative doses of radiation, to face progressive disease several months later in patients who have non-metastatic disease [1, 2]. SBRT became an attractive tool for bringing a solution for recurrent disease by giving high dose radiation to a targeted tumor volume and more durable control while minimizing the dose to OARs, carefully looking for dose constraints and sharp dose fall off associated with SBRT (**Figure 1**) [3].

2. Selection criteria for SBRT: More appropriate patients

The initial research on head and neck SBRT focused on patients who had received high doses of radiation to the head and neck (>30-40 Gy) and experienced recurrent or unresectable lesions. Limited data exists on the utilization of SBRT reirradiation in the postoperative situation. A positive margin, or extensive extra nodal extension [4] metastatic disease and required definitive management [5, 6].

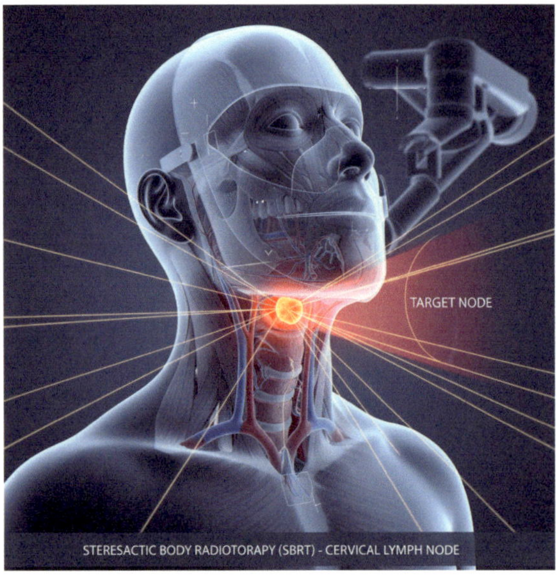

Figure 1.
Multiple radiation beams are targeting a node is shown.

Patients in whom the use of SBRT is more controversial include patients who have resectable recurrent or second primary disease and are medically fit for surgery but refuse an operation for fear of surgical morbidity or other personal preferences (**Figure 2**).

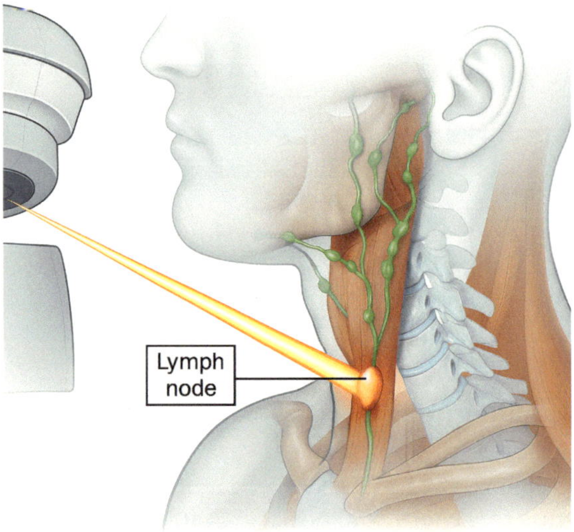

Figure 2.
SBRT is a very precise form of treatment showing the node is targeted without damaging nearby normal structures.

3. Selection criteria for SBRT: Less appropriate patients

3.1 Previously radiated patients

- Resectable recurrent/second primary disease that can be treated
- Gross skin involvement.
- Carotid encasement in link with the lining of the mucosa.
- Widespread disease in the neck (e.g., bilateral or big sized different level of neck node or on the same side.)
- Growth near the spinal cord and brainstem we need to reduce the dose.
- Carcinoma of the larynx/hypopharynx region in the area without previous laryngectomy [7].

3.2 Radiation-naive patients

- Patients who are locally advanced and have non-metastatic head and neck cancer who are eligible for definitive surgery, chemoradiation, or long-course conventional RT
- Patients with extensive metastasis [8].

4. Imaging and target definition

4.1 When doing target definition, the following steps are recommended

1. There should be an oncology committee which should be multidisciplinary between a radiation oncologist, neuroradiologist, and surgical oncologist for target identification while taking into account the detailed history of the patient, including anatomy (which is commonly deformed in the context of recurring illness and the nearby areas for its spread).
2. Collect information from CT scan, PET SCAN, and other imaging modalities.
3. When we are planning with stereotactic body radiation therapy for recurrence in head and neck tumors, we do not frequently electively irradiate nodal levels or delineate a clinical target volume (CTV) margin for treatment of the cancer.
4. Considering the use of modern imaging modalities, we employ GTV to PTV expansion, which is in tune with failing patterns associated with PET/CT-based SBRT.

To preserve typical tissue tolerances in the reirradiation setting, a decreased PTV may be allowed in situations when the PTV margin overlaps with crucial OARs, even though PTV is not strictly defined.

5. Dose fractionation schemes

The literature comprises several dose fractionation schemes. Different types of treatment regimens are primarily conventional, with the oncologist's experience and preference based on the regimen utilized. The radiation dose tolerance of different OARs, including the brain, bone, carotid artery, cranial nerves, skin, and soft tissue, is unknown. The dose-response correlations for recurring malignancies in sites that are previously irradiated tissue with underlying hypoxia and fibrosis remain poorly unexplored [9].

SBRT dose fractionation methods for recurrent head and neck malignancy are still in the research process. To improve drug distribution and alleviate side effects, the majority of centers started fractionating treatments.

A total of five fractions may be categorized as SBRT treatment by CMS. Presently, the majority of US institutions produce doses between 20 and 44 Gy using an aggregate of four to five fractions. Locoregional control was found to be improved in patients who received 40–50 Gy compared to those who received less those that 15–36 Gy.

Tumors having a volume above 25 mL had worse locoregional control than those with volume of 25 mL or less than that. Locoregional control improved in both groups with more of delivered dose. The study examined escalating dosages from 20 to 44 Gy in five sections. Even at the maximum dosage, no grade 3 to 4 or dose-limiting effects were observed [10]. A similar publication by the same group treated some patients with doses of more than 50 Gy.

The University of Pittsburgh group conducted a retrospective study of 70 patients, with 35 (50%) of them. During SBRT treatment, patients received cetuximab infusion. The radiation dose ranged from 40 to 44 Gy, administered in five fractions over five consecutive days. Cetuximab was given at a dose of 400 mg/m^2 1 week before SBRT and 250 mg/m^2 during treatment. Patients receiving cetuximab had a total CR or PR rate of 77.1%, compared to 62.9% in the SBRT-alone group.

6. SBRT for newly diagnosed head and neck cancers

A total of 11 people underwent treatment with SBRT due to various histologies.The dose ranged from 18 Gy in a single fraction to 48 Gy in 16 fractions. A combined CR+ and a partial response rate of 82% was observed, with 1-year local control rate and overall rates of survival of 83 and 70%, respectively. Another study revealed an 84% cumulative response rate in 13 radiation-naive patients who received 35 Gy in five doses [11, 12].

7. Dose to critical structures and toxicity of treatments

Head and neck SBRT has lower overall toxicity than traditional fractionated reirradiation without concurrent systemic treatment. Conventional radiotherapy has elevated incidence of acute grade 3–4 toxicity and treatment-related death, when the use of sophisticated intensity-modulated radiation treatment (IMRT) procedures are used, roughly 5–7%, respectively. SBRT rates are less than 1% at the same endpoints, compared to around 10% for traditional methods. In the aforementioned investigations, cetuximab did not increase toxicity [13].

7.1 Carotid blowout syndrome

CBS is a serious side effect for head and neck cancer patients. The phrase describes the rupture and bleeding of the carotid artery and its main branches. Tumor invasion or harsh treatment-related consequences can lead to branching. CBS can be perplexing. Carotid rupture without uncontrolled illness may indicate a treatment-related issue.

The literature is compounded by a number of uncontrolled disorders that induce rupture. Severe neurological problems are highly prevalent, and death rates vary from 20 to 100%.Carotid artery blowout occurs at a rate of 2.6% following standard reirradiation, with approximately 76% of cases being fatal [14].

After prior exposure, 381 subjects in a Japanese research received five parts with the same average dose of 30 Gy. An 8.4% CBS rate was created by the median RT dose of 60 Gy. This proved fatal to 22 persons. In univariate analysis, older age, skin invasion, and infection signs were revealed as predictors of CBS [15].

In multivariate analysis, skin protrusion was notable. The presence of maceration in the growth, lymph node irradiation, and confirmation of CBS carotid involvement of exceeding 180° by the tumor were found in a matched pair evaluation by an identical group.

In conclusion, the likelihood of a catastrophic carotid arterial blowout may be increased by the following factors [16]:

a. Tumor involving and encasing the artery larger than 180°.

b. Tumor-induced ulceration by involving the mucosa.

c. Skin lesionce tumor.

d. Radiation to draining lymph nodes.

e. Consecutive therapy administration.

To prevent treatment-related mortality, it is very important to carefully identify patients and provide multidisciplinary care if this complication arises. Since thorough dose-volume assessments have not revealed increased toxicity in patients treated with this arrangement, CBS is not regarded by all institutions as a contraindication to SBRT. The carotid dose and CBS are interrelated.

7.2 Spinal cord myelopathy

In investigations on head and neck SBRT, spinal cord myelopathy is infrequent. Two important factors contribute efficiently to this. First is when the initial course of SBRT is delivered, it is important to carefully and precisely plan and limit the maximal dose to lower than 45–50 Gy for the spinal cord. Experiments and clinical data have mentioned that the spinal cord can tolerate reirradiation doses. No neurological toxicity was reported at doses which are less than 18.8 Gy, while doses more than 21.3 Gy resulted in 100% toxicity [17].

In humans, dosages of 5–6 Gy × 5 fractions or 8 Gy × 3 fractions are permissible beyond 30 Gy in 10 fractions at the spinal cord region. The point dose is limited to the utmost allowed quantity (24–30 Gy).

A meta-analysis depicted lower incidence of spinal cord myelopathy with reirradiation at institutions that had given results of their earlier research on spine SBRT experience. Nieder et al. developed risk categorization based on total biologically equivalent dose (BED), interval amongst radiation courses, and one RT treatment with a BED of 102 Gy or above (2 Gy per fraction).

There is significant debate regarding the validity of BED estimates at high exposure percentages and the linear-quadratic (LQ) model. This technique was used by Sahgal et al. to assess spinal cord dose tolerance to reirradiation.

The dose-volume histogram (DVH) of five patients who experienced radiation myelopathy after SBRT reirradiation was compared to that of 14 individuals who did not. They propose the highest possible point dose to the thecal sac for SBRT after previous external beam radiation therapy to the spinal cord [16, 18].

7.3 Brain necrosis

Comparable to those factors mentioned before for spinal cord toxicity, brain necrosis is unusual in SBRT patients. The Quantitative Analyses of Normal Tissue Effects in the Clinic (QUANTEC) proposals gives a complete detailed examination of the dose-volume limits in the brain for both the pre radiated and reirradiation individuals. There were no incidences of brain necrosis when the aggregate BED was below 100 Gy divided into 2 Gy segments.

7.4 Other toxicities

About 100% of patients who get treatment have local incidences of grading 1 and 2 toxicity. Third and fourth grade toxicities are addressed at various tiers, covering acute and late phases. Mucositis, dysphagia, skin or mucosal ulcers, fistula formation, and soft-tissue and damage to bones are examples of serious negative outcomes, also bleeding-out, xerostomia, bleeding, and cranial nerve palsy.

Carotid artery blowout from major blood arteries is the most common cause and immediate cause of death. In recent studies, the use of SBRT for recurring head and neck cancers now results in low or unusual fatality rates.

44 Gy or bigger SBRT doses, provided in five phases on distinct days.

Acute and late toxicity were significantly elevated to grade 3 or higher levels. Patients receiving radiation therapy in the laryngeal/hypopharyngeal area expressed considerably higher acute (20%) and late (50%) morbidity compared to individuals in other head and neck regions [16].

8. Summary of dose constraints

See **Figure 3**.

9. Safety considerations

SBRT's severe hypofractionation and potential for reirradiation toxicity have raised concerns about late toxicity. The incidence of recurrent head and neck cancer has increased.

Some safety measures need to be kept in mind while treating with SBRT.

Unresected Target	8 Gy × 5 < 25 mL 8.8 Gy × 5 > 25 mL
Resected Target (High-risk, Postoperative, and/or + Margins)	**7 Gy × 5**
Critical Structures	**Suggested Dose Limits**
Spinal cord (canal)	24-50 Gy in five fractions maximum
Thecal sac	<15.5 Gy in five fractions
Esophagus	<20-24 Gy in five fractions
Mucosa	<55 Gy EQD_2
Larynx	$D_{5\,mL}$ < 30 Gy
Optic chiasm/nerve	<12 Gy in five fractions
Parotid/salivary	Variable
Mandible	Variable
Carotids	$D_{0.1\,mL}$ < 47.6 Gy *<30 Gy in five fractions*[a]
Brain	<100 Gy BED_2
Skin	<50% prescription dose

Figure 3.
Dose constraints for organs at risk for SBRT.

Reirradiation of head and neck tumors is typically associated with fatal bleeding events, making it a major concern. As mentioned earlier, several clinical variables, including tumors engaging an increased incidence of CBS, have been correlated with the artery bending over 180°, mucosal ulcers, skin damage, nodal irradiation, and therapeutic delivery on consecutive days. Uncontrolled tumors in the head and neck might lead to recurring episodes. Neck cancer poses a high risk of fatal bleeding events. Despite substantial carotid involvement, patients and treating teams may choose to accept the dangers of retreatment.

Organ dysfunction, such as dysphagia and difficulty breathing, is associated with a poor prognosis.

Before considering SBRT, patients with and hypopharynx should be advised of the increased risk of organ dysfunction from reirradiation.

Author details

Shwetima Chaudhary[1*], Abiramasundari V[2] and Vishwadeep Mishra[3]

1 Department of Radiation Oncology, TS Mishra Medical College, Lucknow, India

2 Department of Radiation Oncology, AIIMS Nagpur, Maharashtra, India

3 Department of Radiation Oncology, AIIMS Gorakhpur, Uttar Pradesh, India

*Address all correspondence to: swm222@gmail.com

References

[1] Heron DE, Ferris RL, Karamouzis M, et al. Stereotactic body radiotherapy for recurrent squamous cell carcinoma of the head and neck: Results of a phase I dose-escalation trial. International Journal of Radiation Oncology, Biology, Physics. 2009;**75**:1493-1500. DOI: 10.1016/j.ijrobp.2008.12.075

[2] Vargo JA, Ferris RL, Ohr J, et al. A prospective phase 2 trial of reirradiation with stereotactic body radiation therapy plus cetuximab in patients with previously irradiated recurrent squamous cell carcinoma of the head and neck. International Journal of Radiation Oncology, Biology, Physics. 2015;**91**:480-488. DOI: 10.1016/j.ijrobp.2014.11.023

[3] Vargo JA, Ferris RL, Clump DA, et al. Stereotactic body radiotherapy as primary treatment for elderly patients with medically inoperable head and neck cancer. Frontiers in Oncology. 2014;**4**:214. DOI: 10.3389/fonc.2014.00214

[4] Vargo JA, Kubicek GJ, Ferris RL, et al. Adjuvant stereotactic body radiotherapy ± cetuximab following salvage surgery in previously irradiated head and neck cancer. The Laryngoscope. 2014;**124**:1579-1584. DOI: 10.1002/lary.24441

[5] Fakhry C, Zhang Q, Nguyen-Tan PF, et al. Human papillomavirus and overall survival after progression of oropharyngeal squamous cell carcinoma. Journal of Clinical Oncology. 2014;**32**:3365-3373. DOI: 10.1200/JCO.2014.55.1937

[6] Khan L, Tjong M, Raziee H, et al. Role of stereotactic body radiotherapy for symptom control in head and neck cancer patients. Supportive Care in Cancer. 2015;**23**:1099-1103. DOI: 10.1007/s00520-014-2421-y

[7] Cengiz M, Özyiğit G, Yazici G, et al. Salvage reirradiation with stereotactic body radiotherapy for locally recurrent head-and-neck tumors. International Journal of Radiation Oncology, Biology, Physics. 2011;**81**:104-109. DOI: 10.1016/j.ijrobp.2010.04.027

[8] Yazici G, Sanli TY, Cengiz M, et al. A simple strategy to decrease fatal carotid blowout syndrome after stereotactic body reirradiation for recurrent head and neck cancers. Radiation Oncology. 2013;**8**:242. DOI: 10.1186/1748-717X-8-242

[9] Heron DE, Rwigema JC, Gibson MK, et al. Concurrent cetuximab with stereotactic body radiotherapy for recurrent squamous cell carcinoma of the head and neck: a single-institution matched case-control study. International Journal of Radiation Oncology, Biology, Physics. 2011;**81**(2):e179-e186

[10] Rwigema JC, Heron DE, Ferris RL, et al. The impact of tumor volume and radiotherapy dose on outcome in previously irradiated recurrent squamous cell carcinoma of the head and neck treated with stereotactic body radiation therapy. American Journal of Clinical Oncology. 2011;**34**:372-379. DOI: 10.1097/COC.0b013e3181e84dc0

[11] Siddiqui F, Patel M, Khan M, et al. Stereotactic body radiation therapy for primary, recurrent, and metastatic tumors in the head-and-neck region. International Journal of Radiation Oncology, Biology, Physics. 2009;**74**:1047-1053. DOI: 10.1016/j.ijrobp.2008.09.022

[12] Kodani N, Yamazaki H, Tsubokura T, et al. Stereotactic body radiation therapy for head and neck tumor: Disease control and morbidity outcomes. Journal of Radiation Research. 2011;**52**:24-31

[13] Patel PR, Salama JK. Reirradiation for recurrent head and neck cancer. Expert Review of Anticancer Therapy. 2012;**12**:1177-1189. DOI: 10.1586/era.12.97

[14] Citardi MJ, Chaloupka JC, Son YH, et al. Management of carotid artery rupture by monitored endovascular therapeutic occlusion (1988-1994). The Laryngoscope. 1995;**105**:1086-1092. DOI: 10.1288/00005537-199510000-00015

[15] McDonald MW, Moore MG, Johnstone PA. Risk of carotid blowout after reirradiation of the head and neck: A systematic review. International Journal of Radiation Oncology, Biology, Physics. 2012;**82**:1083-1089. DOI: 10.1016/j.ijrobp.2010.08.029

[16] Vargo JA, Koyfman SA, Ferris RL, Heron DE, Siddiqui F. Head and Neck SBRT. New York (NY): Springer Publishing Company; 2019. ISBN: 9780826168566

[17] Mahadevan A, Floyd S, Wong E, et al. Stereotactic body radiotherapy reirradiation for recurrent epidural spinal metastases. International Journal of Radiation Oncology, Biology, Physics. 2011;**81**:1500-1505. DOI: 10.1016/j.ijrobp.2010.08.012

[18] Kirkpatrick JP, van der Kogel AJ, Schultheiss TE. Radiation dose-volume effects in the spinal cord. International Journal of Radiation Oncology, Biology, Physics. 2010;**76**:S42-S49. DOI: 10.1016/j.ijrobp. 2009.04.095

Chapter 7

Surgical Advances in the Management of Head and Neck Cancer

Liam D. Hyland and Amr Allam

Abstract

This chapter would aim to look at the current surgical advances in the management of head and cancers. This would include TORS (transoral robotic surgery) and TLM (transoral laser microsurgery) being used in oropharyngeal and laryngeal cancers. It would also cover minimally invasive techniques such as use of endoscopic approach for thyroid and parathyroid cancers. The chapter would also look at the advances in reconstructive elements to head and neck cancer management. It would cover development of microvascular free flap reconstruction and perforator flap reconstruction as well as how computer-assisted planning, 3D printing and surgical simulation are increasingly being used to plan complex head and neck cancer reconstructions.

Keywords: TORS, TLM, robotic, endoscopic, minimally invasive, cancer,thyroid, parathyroid, 3D, reconstruction, oncological

1. Introduction

Head and neck cancers encompass a diverse group of malignancies that arise from the oral cavity, pharynx, larynx, thyroid and salivary glands. Over the past two decades, the surgical management of head and neck malignancies has evolved considerably, driven by the pursuit of enhanced precision, reduced morbidity, and improved functional and aesthetic outcomes.

Minimally invasive approaches like Transoral Robotic Surgery (TORS) and Transoral Laser Microsurgery (TLM) have transformed the treatment of tumours in the oropharynx, hypopharynx and larynx. These techniques enable surgeons to access deep anatomical regions via the mouth, thus avoiding external incisions and reducing perioperative morbidity. They provide excellent oncological control while preserving functions of swallow and speech, which is particularly significant in human papillomavirus (HPV) positive oropharyngeal cancers, where organ preservation is a key objective [1, 2].

Parallel advances have taken place in minimally invasive endocrine surgery, with the introduction of remote-access and endoscopic techniques that prioritise cosmesis and recovery without compromising safety. Procedures such as minimally invasive video-assisted thyroidectomy (MIVAT) and the transoral endoscopic thyroidectomy vestibular approach (TOETVA) offer a swifter recovery and reduced pain, while imaging-guided parathyroidectomy provides excellent cure rates [3, 4].

In reconstructive surgery, the refinement of free tissue transfer and perforator flap techniques has improved functional and aesthetic outcomes following oncological resection. Harvesting options such as fibula, radial forearm and anterolateral thigh flaps provide tailored reconstruction of bone and soft tissue, while advances in flap monitoring and surgical workflow have further optimised success rates [5, 6].

Computer-assisted planning and three-dimensional (3D) technologies have also enhanced surgical precision and predictability. Virtual surgical planning (VSP), 3D printing and intraoperative navigation now allow for personalised multidisciplinary care, particularly in complex skull base and midface procedures [7–9].

This chapter will examine each of these domains in detail, starting with transoral approaches that have redefined access to deep anatomical regions through minimally invasive techniques. It will then explore the latest innovations in endocrine surgery, where remote-access and scarless procedures are transforming thyroid and parathyroid management. Building on these advances, the chapter will then look at reconstructive strategies, including microvascular and perforator flap techniques, that restore both function and form following ablative surgery. Finally, it will consider how digital planning and three-dimensional (3D) technologies are reshaping surgical precision and simulation, marking a new frontier in head and neck oncological care.

2. Transoral surgical techniques

2.1 Transoral robotic surgery (TORS)

Transoral Robotic Surgery (TORS) allows minimally invasive resection of tumours of the oropharynx through the oral cavity using robotic instrumentation, avoiding the morbidity associated with mandibulotomy and pharyngotomy. The system incorporates a high-definition 3D camera and wristed instruments mounted on robotic arms which are controlled remotely by a surgeon. This setup offers enhanced visualisation and dexterity, allowing precise dissection in anatomically confined regions [10, 11].

TORS is particularly advantageous for tumours within the oropharynx of which the subsites include the tonsillar complex, base of tongue and posterior oropharyngeal wall. It has been associated with shorter hospital stays, reduced need for tracheostomy and faster resumption of oral intake when compared with open approaches [12]. Functional outcomes, including swallowing and speech, are also superior, with lower gastrostomy and tracheostomy dependence reported. Importantly, TORS permits accurate pathological staging, enabling personalised adjuvant therapy which is especially relevant for HPV positive oropharyngeal squamous cell carcinoma (SCC) where treatment de-escalation is under active investigation [13].

Clinical evidence supports the oncological efficacy of TORS; a large retrospective cohort study of 184 patients with HPV positive oropharyngeal SCC reported a five-year disease-specific survival of 94.4% with low recurrence rates [14]. Trials such as ECOG 3311 and PATHOS demonstrate that histopathological staging after TORS can guide tailored adjuvant therapy, potentially reducing radiation exposure without compromising outcomes [15, 16].

Functional preservation is also a major benefit as seen when compared with other treatment modalities such as chemoradiation. TORS patients show lower gastrostomy dependence and better swallowing outcomes at 1 year [12].

These advantages are particularly relevant in younger HPV positive patients where long-term quality of life is paramount.

However, there are a number of limitations associated with TORS. Adequate oropharyngeal exposure is essential, and so anatomical constraints such as trismus or retrognathia may preclude safe access. Robotic systems are also costly and require specialised training; credentialing pathways and simulation-based education are increasingly employed to standardise safe implementation [17].

In summary, TORS represents a paradigm shift in the management of oropharyngeal SCC, offering strong oncological outcomes with superior functional preservation. Its role is expanding as evidence for treatment de-escalation grows, consolidating its place in the multidisciplinary care of HPV associated cancers.

2.2 Transoral laser microsurgery (TLM)

Transoral Laser Microsurgery (TLM) uses a carbon dioxide (CO_2) laser coupled with a microlaryngoscope to excise tumours through the mouth without external incisions. The technique offers fine dissection under microscopic guidance, enabling accurate tumour removal while sparing surrounding structures critical for speech and swallowing [18, 19].

TLM is particularly valuable for early stage glottic and supraglottic cancers where voice preservation is a priority. Like TORS, it is associated with low complication rates, minimal bleeding and reduced gastrostomy dependence compared with chemoradiation [20]. Outcomes are generally superior in terms of swallowing and voice quality while avoiding radiation-induced fibrosis and xerostomia [21].

Oncological results are robust; local control for T1 glottic cancers treated with TLM reaches 85–95% with five-year disease-specific survival rates exceeding 90% in most series [22]. TLM is also repeatable, making it effective in salvage settings where radiorecurrent disease might otherwise require laryngectomy [22, 23].

Functional results in supraglottic cancers are similarly favourable with lower gastrostomy and tracheostomy rates compared with radiotherapy [24]. While aspiration risk remains a concern, careful patient selection and rehabilitation can help to minimise this. The technique can also be combined with neck dissection when indicated, ensuring comprehensive oncological management.

Limitations include the requirement for excellent laryngeal exposure which may be restricted by cervical spine rigidity or limited mouth opening. The steep learning curve in mastering laser physics and endoscopic technique also restricts availability. Centres with high TLM expertise consistently report better outcomes, highlighting the importance of surgical training and institutional support [19].

In summary, TLM remains a cornerstone in the management of early stage glottic carcinoma, balancing oncological efficacy with functional preservation. Its repeatability and organ-preserving nature make it an essential component of minimally invasive head and neck surgery.

3. Minimally invasive endocrine surgery

3.1 Endoscopic thyroidectomy

Endoscopic thyroidectomy enables removal of all or part of the thyroid through small remote incisions using an endoscope, thereby avoiding a visible anterior neck scar. Approaches include the transaxillary, retroauricular and transoral vestibular routes. These provide superior cosmetic outcomes while reducing tissue disruption. High-definition cameras and CO_2 insufflation enhance the surgical field, and robotic assistance improves precision and ergonomics in complex cases [25, 26].

The transoral endoscopic thyroidectomy vestibular approach (TOETVA) has gained prominence for producing a truly scarless outcome; accessing the thyroid via the oral vestibule, TOETVA aligns with natural orifice transluminal endoscopic surgery (NOTES). Clinical studies confirm its safety in selected patients, with complication rates comparable to open thyroidectomy, though it requires meticulous skill to avoid mental nerve injury [27].

The minimally invasive video-assisted thyroidectomy (MIVAT) remains a widely used method for small benign nodules and low-risk malignancies. Using a central incision under 2.5 cm, MIVAT provides reduced pain, faster recovery and improved cosmetic satisfaction compared with open surgery [28]. Remote-access approaches such as transaxillary and retroauricular thyroidectomy are also viable options for patients seeking to avoid visible scars. These require more extensive dissection and longer operating times but can be facilitated by robotic systems which improve instrument manoeuvrability [29].

Despite their advantages, not all patients are suitable candidates for these methods. Contraindications include large goitres, substernal extension, previous neck surgery and locally invasive disease. In addition, both TOETVA and robotic approaches involve steep learning curves and demand dedicated training. As these techniques mature, ongoing research will be critical in refining indications and optimising outcomes [30].

3.2 Parathyroid surgery

Minimally invasive parathyroidectomy (MIP) has become the standard for treating primary hyperparathyroidism in patients with concordant preoperative localisation. Unlike traditional bilateral neck exploration, MIP uses targeted approaches based on imaging, most commonly sestamibi scans and high-resolution ultrasound, to identify the adenomatous gland. A small, focussed incision reduces operative time, postoperative pain and hospital stay [31, 32].

The use of intraoperative parathyroid hormone (PTH) monitoring, often guided by the Miami criterion (>50% PTH drop post-excision), helps to confirm cure and reduces the risk of persistent disease. With accurate imaging and PTH monitoring, MIP achieves cure rates exceeding 95% while minimising morbidity [33].

Endoscopic and robotic techniques are also applied in selected parathyroid cases, particularly bilateral disease, revision surgery or patients with strong cosmetic concerns. Remote-access approaches via the axilla or oral vestibule have shown promising results, though they remain less common than standard MIP [34].

Endoscopic parathyroidectomy offers rapid recovery, minimal dissection and high patient satisfaction. Intraoperative nerve monitoring is routinely employed to protect the recurrent laryngeal nerve, further improving safety. High-volume centres consistently report excellent outcomes, reinforcing the value of experience and institutional expertise [35].

In summary, minimally invasive thyroid and parathyroid surgery now provide effective, cosmetically favourable alternatives to open surgery, offering excellent outcomes when patients are carefully selected. The integration of endoscopic, robotic and imaging-guided strategies continues to expand the boundaries of endocrine surgery.

4. Advances in reconstructive surgery

4.1 Microvascular free flap reconstruction

Microvascular free flap reconstruction remains the gold standard for restoring complex head and neck defects after oncological resection. These flaps provide vascularised tissue capable of replacing bone, muscle and mucosa, allowing both functional and aesthetic rehabilitation. Common donor sites include the fibula free flap for osseous reconstruction, the radial forearm free flap (RFFF) for intraoral lining, and the anterolateral thigh (ALT) flap for bulk soft tissue replacement [36].

The fibula flap is particularly suited to mandibular reconstruction due to its robust cortical bone, long pedicle and compatibility with dental implants. It can be osteotomised to recreate mandibular contour and skin paddles allow simultaneous repair of mucosal or cutaneous defects [37].

The RFFF, long regarded as a workhorse flap, offers thin, pliable tissue ideal for intraoral or pharyngeal defects with reliable vascular anatomy facilitating harvest. Donor site morbidity such as sensory changes and cold intolerance, remains a limitation, prompting use of alternatives in younger or highly active patients [38].

The ALT flap provides versatility with its variable thickness, long pedicle and large harvestable skin area. It is used for through-and-through defects, skull base reconstruction and total glossectomy. The ability to thin or bulk the flap intraoperatively adds further flexibility [39].

Advances in monitoring techniques such as implantable Doppler probes, near-infrared spectroscopy and thermal imaging have improved flap survival by enabling early detection of vascular compromise. The two-team approach, in which one team performs tumour ablation while the other harvests the flap, reduces operating times and anaesthetic exposure which subsequently improves outcomes especially in elderly or comorbid patients [40].

While highly effective, free flap surgery demands significant microsurgical expertise and postoperative support. Outcomes are consistently superior in high-volume centres. Increasing integration with computer-assisted planning and 3D modelling is further enhancing accuracy in flap design and inset [41].

4.2 Perforator flap techniques

Perforator flaps represent a refinement of free tissue transfer, using skin and subcutaneous tissue supplied by perforating vessels while sparing underlying muscle. This reduces donor site morbidity while maintaining vascular reliability. Commonly used examples in head and neck reconstruction include the ALT perforator flap and the medial sural artery perforator (MSAP) flap [42].

The ALT perforator flap provides a large harvestable skin paddle, long pedicle and adjustable thickness, making it suitable for subtotal glossectomy, buccal mucosa and orbitomaxillary defects. Suprafascial harvest allows creation of a thinner flap when required and donor site morbidity is minimal with frequent primary closure [39].

The MSAP flap is particularly useful for small to medium intraoral defects in patients unsuitable for radial forearm harvest. It provides thin, pliable tissue with favourable contouring properties and reduced donor site complications. Comparative studies suggest that functional outcomes and survival rates are equivalent to RFFF but with improved donor site satisfaction [42].

Preoperative imaging with Doppler ultrasound, CT angiography or thermal mapping optimises perforator selection and thus reduces intraoperative uncertainty. Emerging augmented reality (AR) tools are being trialled to visualise perforator anatomy intraoperatively [41].

Supermicrosurgery, involving anastomosis of vessels ≤0.8 mm, has expanded the role of perforator flaps. It allows for perforator-to-perforator connections which are useful in patients with compromised axial vessels due to prior surgery or radiotherapy [43].

Perforator flaps are particularly valuable for facial and intraoral reconstructions where thin, mobile tissue is essential for speech and swallowing. Their pliability permits functional and aesthetic reconstructions that better integrate with surrounding tissues [42].

While outcomes are excellent, perforator flap surgery requires advanced microsurgical skill and familiarity with anatomical variation. As imaging and supermicrosurgical techniques evolve, perforator flaps are expected to become increasingly essential for patient-tailored reconstruction [44].

5. Computer-assisted planning and 3D technologies

5.1 Virtual surgical planning (VSP)

Virtual surgical planning (VSP) integrates CT or magnetic resonance imaging (MRI) imaging with computer-aided design (CAD) software to simulate resections and reconstructions. This protocol allows surgeons to anticipate challenges, plan osteotomies with millimetric precision, and achieve better symmetry and contour. VSP is especially valuable in mandibular and midface reconstruction where restoration of occlusion and aesthetics is critical [45].

In fibula free flap reconstructions, VSP supports simultaneous planning of bone orientation and dental implant placement, enabling immediate dental rehabilitation. Integration with digital dentistry has further improved functional outcomes [46]. Comparative studies show that VSP-guided reconstructions reduce operative time and complications relative to freehand techniques [47].

While highly effective, VSP requires access to specialised software, advanced imaging and engineering collaboration, all of which may limit adoption in resource-constrained centres. Wider access to open-source platforms is beginning to address these challenges [45].

5.2 3D printing

Three-dimensional (3D) printing has become an indispensable adjunct to planning and executing complex reconstructions. Anatomical models, cutting guides and implants can be fabricated from imaging data, providing tactile references and improving surgical accuracy.

In-house 3D printing allows rapid production of models and guides, reducing delays in time-sensitive oncology cases [8]. Cutting guides derived from VSP ensure precise osteotomies and alignment which can improve both functional and cosmetic outcomes [47].

Custom implants, including titanium plates and prosthetic components, can be produced to match patient-specific anatomy. Preoperative fabrication reduces intraoperative contouring and implant-related complications [8]. Beyond planning,

3D-printed models also provide excellent educational tools for both surgeons in training and patients undergoing treatment.

5.3 Surgical simulation and navigation

Surgical simulation using virtual reality (VR) and augmented reality (AR) is transforming surgical training and preoperative preparation. Immersive simulations allow for the development of technical skills and improved spatial awareness without risk to patients. Patient-specific digital models offer realistic practice and assessment of competence [9].

Intraoperative navigation systems use preoperative imaging data to provide real-time feedback which can enhance accuracy and safety. They are particularly useful in skull base and orbital surgery, where avoiding critical neurovascular structures is paramount [47].

AR overlays provide intraoperative visualisation of tumour margins, vascular anatomy and osteotomies. Studies show AR-assisted surgery improves margin control and reduces operative time, particularly when combined with navigation and 3D-printed guides [45].

VR, AR and navigation technologies are enhancing both surgical training and intraoperative performance, supporting the move towards more personalised and precise oncological care [45].

6. Conclusion

The past two decades have witnessed a paradigm shift in the surgical management of head and neck cancers. Minimally invasive transoral techniques such as TORS and TLM have expanded access to deep anatomical sites while preserving function, particularly in HPV related disease. Additionally, scarless endocrine approaches, including TOETVA and MIVAT, have redefined cosmetic outcomes and recovery profiles without compromising oncological safety. Advances in reconstructive surgery, particularly microvascular and perforator flaps, have further transformed survivorship by restoring both form and function, while continuous refinements in flap monitoring and surgical workflow have improved predictability and safety. Equally transformative are the digital tools now entering routine practice; VSP, 3D printing and immersive simulation technologies are no longer experimental luxuries but integral components of personalised care.

Together, these innovations represent a new surgical era: one defined not by choosing between oncological control and quality of life, but by striving for both. As techniques mature and technology becomes more accessible, the future of head and neck oncological surgery will be increasingly precise, less invasive and more patient-centred. The challenge for the next generation of surgeons is not simply to adopt these advances but to continue pushing their boundaries, ensuring that innovation consistently translates into longer survival and restored function.

Author details

Liam D. Hyland[1*] and Amr Allam[2]

1 ENT CT2, Queen's Medical Centre, Nottingham, UK

2 Advanced Head and Neck Surgical Oncology Fellow, Queen's Medical Centre, Nottingham, UK

*Address all correspondence to: liamhyland1996@gmail.com

IntechOpen

References

[1] Dziegielewski PT et al. Transoral robotic surgery for oropharyngeal cancer. JAMA Otolaryngology–Head & Neck Surgery. 2013;**139**(11):1099. DOI: 10.1001/jamaoto.2013.2747

[2] Weinstein GS et al. Transoral robotic surgery. Archives of Otolaryngology–Head & Neck Surgery. 2007;**133**(12):1220. DOI: 10.1001/archotol.133.12.1220

[3] Moore EJ et al. Transoral robotic surgery for oropharyngeal carcinoma: Surgical margins and oncologic outcomes. Head & Neck. 2018;**40**(4): 747-755. DOI: 10.1002/hed.25055

[4] de Almeida JR et al. Oncologic outcomes after transoral robotic surgery. JAMA Otolaryngology–Head & Neck Surgery. 2015;**141**(12):1043. DOI: 10.1001/jamaoto.2015.1508

[5] Tsang R. Review for 'swallowing outcomes after transoral robotic surgery and adjuvant treatment in unknown primary [Preprint]. 2024. DOI: 10.1111/odi.15063/v1/review2

[6] Ferris RL et al. Phase II randomized trial of transoral surgery and low-dose intensity modulated radiation therapy in resectable P16+ locally advanced oropharynx cancer: An ECOG-acrin cancer research group trial (E3311). Journal of Clinical Oncology. 2022;**40**(2):138-149. DOI: 10.1200/jco.21.01752

[7] Ganesh PS, Pathoor NN, Gopal RK. Reflection on transoral robotic surgery vs transoral laser microsurgery in HPV-positive oropharyngeal squamous cell carcinoma. JAMA Otolaryngology–Head & Neck Surgery. 2025;**151**(4):413. DOI: 10.1001/jamaoto.2024.5061

[8] Sethi RKV, Chen MM, Malloy KM. Complications of transoral robotic surgery. Otolaryngologic Clinics of North America. 2020;**53**(6):1109-1115. DOI: 10.1016/j.otc.2020.07.017

[9] Canis M et al. Organ preservation in T4A laryngeal cancer: Is transoral laser microsurgery an option? European Archives of Oto-Rhino-Laryngology. 2013;**270**(10):2719-2727. DOI: 10.1007/s00405-013-2382-7

[10] Peretti G et al. Transoral laser microsurgery as primary treatment for selected T3 glottic and supraglottic cancers. Head & Neck. 2016;**38**(7): 1107-1112. DOI: 10.1002/hed.24424

[11] Meulemans J et al. Transoral laser microsurgery (TLM) for glottic cancer: Prospective assessment of a new pathology workup protocol. Frontiers in Surgery. 2020;**7**. DOI: 10.3389/fsurg.2020.00056

[12] Lee HS et al. Voice outcome according to surgical extent of transoral laser microsurgery for T1 glottic carcinoma. The Laryngoscope. 2015;**126**(9):2051-2056. DOI: 10.1002/lary.25789

[13] Anuwong A et al. Transoral endoscopic thyroidectomy vestibular approach (TOETVA): Indications, techniques and results. Surgical Endoscopy. 2017;**32**(1):456-465. DOI: 10.1007/s00464-017-5705-8

[14] Razavi CR, Russell JO. Indications and contraindications to transoral thyroidectomy. Annals of Thyroid. 2017;**2**:12-12. DOI: 10.21037/aot.2017.10.01

[15] Miccoli P, Minuto MN. Minimally invasive video-assisted

parathyroidectomy (MIVAP) and minimally invasive video-assisted thyroidectomy (MIVAT). In: Innovations in Modern Endocrine Surgery. 2021. pp. 235-243. DOI: 10.1007/978-3-030-73951-5_17

[16] Gupta A. Transoral endoscopic thyroidectomy vestibular approach (TOETVA). Transoral Endoscopic Thyroidectomy Vestibular Approach (TOETVA). 2024;**1**(1):105-106. DOI: 10.62830/mmj1-4-18c

[17] Udelsman R, Lin Z, Donovan P. The superiority of minimally invasive parathyroidectomy based on 1650 consecutive patients with primary hyperparathyroidism. Annals of Surgery. 2011;**253**(3):585-591. DOI: 10.1097/sla.0b013e318208fed9

[18] Irvin GL, Solorzano CC, Carneiro DM. Quick intraoperative parathyroid hormone assay: Surgical adjunct to allow limited parathyroidectomy, improve success rate, and predict outcome. World Journal of Surgery. 2004;**28**(12):1287-1292. DOI: 10.1007/s00268-004-7708-6

[19] Kwon RJ. Minimally invasive parathyroidectomy versus conventional surgery for primary hyperparathyroidism. Oxford Medicine Online [Preprint]. 2017. DOI: 10.1093/med/9780199384075.003.0043

[20] Okoh AK, Sound S, Berber E. Robotic parathyroidectomy. Journal of Surgical Oncology. 2015;**112**(3):240-242. DOI: 10.1002/jso.23911

[21] Wenig BL, Keller AJ. Microvascular free flap reconstruction for head and neck defects. Archives of Otolaryngology - Head and Neck Surgery. 1989;**115**(9):1118-1120. DOI: 10.1001/archotol.1989.01860330108029

[22] Hidalgo DA. Aesthetic improvements in free-flap mandible reconstruction. Plastic and Reconstructive Surgery. 1991;**88**(4):574-585. DOI: 10.1097/00006534-199110000-00003

[23] Wei F-C et al. Fibula osteoseptocutaneous flap for reconstruction of composite mandibular defects. Plastic and Reconstructive Surgery. 1994;**93**(2):294-304. DOI: 10.1097/00006534-199402000-00009

[24] Hanasono MM et al. Success of sequential free flaps in head and neck reconstruction. Journal of Plastic, Reconstructive & Aesthetic Surgery. 2014;**67**(9):1186-1193. DOI: 10.1016/j.bjps.2014.05.012

[25] Yu P. Reinnervated anterolateral thigh flap for tongue reconstruction. Head & Neck. 2004;**26**(12):1038-1044. DOI: 10.1002/hed.20106

[26] Grotting JC. Free flap monitoring: A review of current practice. Microsurgery. 1995;**16**(11):727-727. DOI: 10.1002/micr.1920161104

[27] Hanasono MM et al. Midfacial reconstruction using virtual planning, rapid prototype modeling, and stereotactic navigation. Plastic and Reconstructive Surgery. 2010;**126**(6):2002-2006. DOI: 10.1097/prs.0b013e3181f447e1

[28] Kim JT. Contribution of perforator flaps in the flap selection for head and neck reconstruction. Korean Society for Head and Neck Oncology. 2019;**35**(1):1-11. DOI: 10.21593/kjhno/2019.35.1.1

[29] Mathur BS, Pappalardo M. Tongue reconstruction with medial sural artery perforator flap. In: Clinical Scenarios in Reconstructive

Microsurgery. 2022. pp. 99-108. DOI: 10.1007/978-3-030-23706-6_12

[30] Ciudad P et al. The radial forearm free flap as a "vascular bridge" for secondary microsurgical head and neck reconstruction in a vessel-depleted neck. Microsurgery. 2017;**38**(6):651-658. DOI: 10.1002/micr.30259

[31] Saint-Cyr M et al. The perforasome theory: Vascular anatomy and clinical implications. Plastic and Reconstructive Surgery. 2009;**124**(5):1529-1544. DOI: 10.1097/prs.0b013e3181b98a6c

[32] Su Y et al. Editorial: Virtual surgical planning and 3D printing in head and neck tumor resection and reconstruction. Frontiers in Oncology. 2022;**12**. DOI: 10.3389/fonc.2022.960545

[33] Dean A et al. Fibula free flap in maxillomandibular reconstruction. Factors related to osteosynthesis plates' complications. Journal of Cranio-Maxillofacial Surgery. 2020;**48**(10):994-1003. DOI: 10.1016/j.jcms.2020.08.003

[34] Sharaf BA et al. Virtual surgical planning in craniomaxillofacial surgery: A systematic review and meta-analysis of accuracy, operative time, and cost-effectiveness. Journal of Plastic, Reconstructive & Aesthetic Surgery. 2025;**105**:305-314. DOI: 10.1016/j.bjps.2025.04.037

[35] Reuther JF, Meier JL. Microvascular surgical tissue transfer for reconstruction in the head and neck area. Oral and Maxillofacial Surgery Clinics of North America. 1993;**5**(4):687-710. DOI: 10.1016/s1042-3699(20)307299

[36] Manzie T. AI-driven biomechanical virtual surgical planning for optimized jaw reconstruction. British Journal of Oral and Maxillofacial Surgery. 2025;**63**(10). DOI: 10.1016/j.bjoms.2025.09.161

[37] Ettinger KS et al. Patient-specific implants improve volumetric surgical accuracy compared to stock reconstruction plates in modern paradigm virtual surgical planning of fibular free flaps for head and neck reconstruction. Journal of Oral and Maxillofacial Surgery. 2024;**82**(10):1311-1328. DOI: 10.1016/j.joms.2024.06.166

[38] Isikay I et al. Narrative review of patient-specific 3D visualization and reality technologies in skull base neurosurgery: Enhancements in surgical training, planning, and navigation. Frontiers in Surgery. 2024;**11**. DOI: 10.3389/fsurg.2024.1427844

[39] Dirven S, Allen JE. Physical and virtual modelling of the head and neck for surgical simulation and training. Current Opinion in Otolaryngology & Head and Neck Surgery. 2016;**24**(6):463-468. DOI: 10.1097/moo.0000000000000303

[40] Probst FA et al. Computer-assisted designed and manufactured procedures facilitate the lingual application of mandible reconstruction plates. Journal of Oral and Maxillofacial Surgery. 2016;**74**(9):1879-1895. DOI: 10.1016/j.joms.2016.03.015

[41] Hanasono MM, Matros E, Disa JJ. Important aspects of head and neck reconstruction. Plastic and Reconstructive Surgery. 2014;**134**(6). DOI: 10.1097/prs.0000000000000722

[42] Roser SM et al. The accuracy of virtual surgical planning in free fibula mandibular reconstruction: Comparison of planned and final results. Journal of Oral and Maxillofacial Surgery. 2010;**68**(11):2824-2832. DOI: 10.1016/j.joms.2010.06.177

[43] Gander T et al. Patient specific implants (PSI) in reconstruction of orbital floor and wall fractures. Journal of Cranio-Maxillofacial Surgery. 2015;**43**(1):126-130. DOI: 10.1016/j.jcms.2014.10.024

[44] Rosu S et al. O.265 computer assisted tridimensional facial reconstruction. Journal of Cranio-Maxillofacial Surgery. 2008;**36**. DOI: 10.1016/s1010-5182(08)71389-1

[45] Hassfeld S et al. Preoperative planning and intraoperative navigation in skull base surgery. Journal of Cranio-Maxillofacial Surgery. 1998;**26**(4):220-225. DOI: 10.1016/s1010-5182(98)80017-6

[46] Werker PMN. Microsurgical reconstruction of the head and neck. Journal of Plastic, Reconstructive & Aesthetic Surgery. 2010;**63**(5):885. DOI: 10.1016/j.bjps.2010.01.031

[47] El-Maghraby H et al. A prospective study to evaluate the efficacy of frameless, pinless electromagnetic image-guided navigation in endoscopic skull base surgery. Journal of Neurological Surgery Part B: Skull Base. 2012;**73**(S02). DOI: 10.1055/s-0032-1314333

Chapter 8

Systemic Therapies for Relapse/ Metastatic Head and Neck Squamous Cell Carcinoma

Andrea Alberti

Abstract

Treatment of patients with relapse/metastatic head and neck cancer has evolved significantly over the past 20 years with new therapeutic opportunities that have changed the natural history of these patients. From the efficacy data of single-dose chemotherapy drugs, we have come to define the best chemotherapy backbone in this category of patients. The Extreme and Tpex studies introduced the monoclonal anti-EGFR antibody cetuximab in the frontline. Subsequently, Keynote 048 and Checkmate 141 introduced immunotherapy with checkpoint inhibitor drugs (ICI) into daily practice, increasing the spectrum of therapeutic options for these patients. The introduction of ICI at earlier stages of treatment has also improved the activity and efficacy of subsequent lines of therapy, increasing the complexity of treatment flowcharts. This chapter retraces the steps that have led to the definition of the current therapeutic path in patients with R/M HNSCC, highlighting the activity of the drugs and their combination, prognostic expectations and safety data.

Keywords: chemotherapy, cetuximab, pembrolizumab, therapeutic strategy, treatment activity, patient's prognosis

1. Introduction

At the time of diagnosis of head and neck squamous cell carcinoma (HNSCC), only 4–12% of all patients have already a metastatic disease [1]. However, the locoregional or metastatic relapse of disease, following a curative and radical treatment, affects about 20% of patients with primary diagnosis of early stage HNSCC and up to 50% of patients with diagnostic findings of locally advanced HNSCC [2]. At diagnosis of recurrent and/or metastatic HNSCC (R/M HNSCC), the therapeutic possibilities to be pursued depend on the previously treatment, the clinical and frailty characteristics of the patient and based on the tumor site. It should be noted that, in this disease setting, there may still be a chance for a radical treatment. For selected patients, with oligometastatic disease at diagnosis, it is still possible to consider salvage resection, re-irradiation [3] or metastatectomy (particularly for HPV-positive cancer) [4] that has curative purpose. In contrast, when the loco-regional disease is not manageable with surgery or radiotherapy, when presence of several distant metastatic nodes or a short disease-free interval with a high growing relapse (aggressive biological behavior), absolute priority is given to the initiation of palliative systemic treatment [5]. The purpose of active oncological treatment is to relieve symptoms, improve quality of life and prolong survival. Therefore, the primary objectives are clinical efficacy measured by the overall survival (OS), and secondary the clinical activity measured as overall response rate (ORR) and progression free survival (PFS).

The following paragraph intends to retrace the systemic treatments with palliative intention that, over time, have consolidated as therapeutic lines for R/M HNSCC.

2. First outcomes of chemotherapy regimens

Since the 1980s, platinum-based chemotherapy has been a milestone in the treatment of R/M HNSCC. Two studies demonstrated the efficacy of systemic monotherapy with cisplatin than other chemotherapy drugs. The phase III trial conducted by Morton et al. showed a significant increase in OS of platinum monotherapy than Bleomycin with an ORR of 25% [6]. In a subsequent phase III study, 200 patients were randomized to receive one of the following regimens: cisplatin alone, methotrexate alone, cisplatin +5FU or cisplatin + methotrexate. The patients treated with cisplatin had a significantly longer OS than patients treated with methotrexate monotherapy, with an OS of 7.3 and 4.3 months ($p < 0.025$), respectively and an ORR of 21% [7].

Therefore, when the efficacy of cisplatin in monotherapy was established, the second step was to understand whether the combination of cisplatin plus other cytotoxic drugs could further improve results of active oncological treatments. Kish et al. presented encouraging results of the association of cisplatin plus 5-FU with an ORR of 70% with 27% of complete responses. This study showed, therefore, that the combination of Cisplatin +5-FU had an advantage in terms of tumor response, dependent on the patient performance status and comorbidities. In patients with optimal performance status the ORR reached 70%, whereas in patients with sub-optimal performance status the ORR was around 33% [8]. Furthermore, from later series of randomized phase III trials the cisplatin-based combination regimens resulted more active in term of ORR than monotherapy, without any advantage in OS. These clinical trials compared platinum (cisplatin and carboplatin) and 5-FU as monotherapy or in combination with paclitaxel and pemetrexed [9–12]. The results were agreed to show that, in platinum-based combination schemes, the ORR was quite 32%, significantly higher than single agent monotherapy regimens of cisplatin (ORR 9–17% [9, 12]), 5-FU (ORR 13% [9]) and Methotrexate (ORR 10% [10]). In cisplatin-combined regimens, however, treatment-related toxicity also increased, without showing any advantage on patients' OS compared to monotherapy regimens.

Apart to the platinum-based regimens, single-arm phase two trials explore the activity of other mono-chemotherapy regimens, like pemetrexed, docetaxel, paclitaxel, gemcitabine, capecitabine, irinotecan, vinorelbine and ixabepilone [13]. The monotherapies that showed the greatest benefit in terms of ORR and OS were paclitaxel with 36–40% and median OS of 9.2 month [14, 15], Docetaxel with 20–42% ORR and median OS of 6.7 months [16–18], Capecitabine with 24% ORR and median OS of 7.3 months [19] and Pemetrexed with 26% ORR and median OS of 7.3 months [20]. The optimal treatment of elderly subjects with R/M HNSCC cannot be separated from a careful evaluation of the patients' clinical characteristics, since many of them have medical comorbidities, poor performance status and lack of psycho-social support. Argiris et al. reported evidence from two phase III studies, conducted by the Eastern Cooperative Oncology Group (ECOG) on R/M HNSCC, involving elderly patients (aged 70 years) treated in line with combination chemotherapy regimens, all containing cisplatin and a second cytotoxic drug (5-FU or Paclitaxel). The median OS did not differ between elderly and young patients, but older patients had higher treatment-related toxicity and a tendency for a higher rate of treatment-related deaths [21]. Although some elderly patients, appropriately selected on the basis of an optimal performance status and an acceptable fragility index, could tolerate double platinum therapy, for the majority of the population aged over 70, monotherapy regimens associated with supportive care were more appropriate, not less effective but with a more acceptable toxicity profile [13]. In conclusion, compared to single-agent protocols, platinum-based combination regimens lead to a beneficial increase in ORR but without significantly improving patients' overall survival and with a higher rate of adverse events in terms of nausea, vomiting, nephropathy and hematologic toxicity [7, 22]. Based on this evidence the combination of platinum plus 5FU has been adopted as standard of care for R/M HNSCC. The increased activity of this combination could significantly benefit patients with symptoms related to the burden of disease, for whom the benefit of a tumor response could be such as to justify treatment-related toxicity. In contrast, for patients with low disease load and no symptoms associated with the tumor, a monotherapy with cisplatin, pemetrexed, methotrexate, capecitabine, paclitaxel or docetaxel could be indicated with a less severe toxicity profile [13].

Later trials demonstrated cetuximab (anti-EGFR monoclonal antibody) activity in patients resistant to platinum chemotherapy. Two single arm phase II trials, published in 2005 and conducted by Baselga et al. and Herbst et al., enrolled patients who had experienced progression disease or stable disease to a previous platinum-based chemotherapy regimen [23, 24]. In this refractory setting, the addition of cetuximab to cisplatin was tested. The evidence suggested that for patients with platinum-refractory R/M HNSCC (characterized by poor prognosis), the addiction of cetuximab to cisplatinum chemotherapy resulted able to revert progression, achieving an ORR of 10–13%, with a median OS of 6.5 months [23, 24]. These low response rate suggested that the benefits were due to the activity of cetuximab and not its combination with platinum-based chemotherapy. In addition, the administration of cetuximab was not shown to exacerbate platinum-related toxicity but was associated with adverse skin effects and allergic infusion reactions [23]. This led to a clinical trial to assess the benefits and tolerability of cetuximab as a single agent in patients with R/M HNSCC who had experienced progression to standard platinum-based chemotherapy. Vermorken et al. published in 2007 the results of this phase II study, in line with those obtained from the previous combination, the ORR was 13%, the disease control rate (DCR) was 46%, the median time to progression was 2.3 months, while OS was 178 days. Treatment with cetuximab alone was well tolerated and, again in this context, the main toxicity emerged as skin rash and allergic reactions at infusion [25].

3. The EXTREME combination regime for platinum-sensitive R/M HNSCC, shows an increase in overall survival

Head-neck cancers often exhibit oncogenic dependence on EGFR and this contributes to worsening their prognosis. The previous evidence of significant activity of cetuximab in platinum-resistant R/M HNSCC forms and its acceptable tolerability profile supported the testing of this monoclonal anti-antibody EGFR, in combination with standard of care chemotherapy, as the first line for R/M HNSCC [26, 27]. The evidence was encouraging, in particular, the phase III randomized clinical trial conducted by Burtness et al. reported a significant increase in overall tumor response in the group treated with Cisplatin + Cetuximab, with an ORR of 26%, compared to patients treated with cisplatin alone, whose ORR was 10% ($p = 0.03$). Although not statistically significant, the arm treated with Cetuximab experienced a better median OS of 9.2 months, even chemotherapy alone achieved a median OS of 8 months. Interesting, patients who developed dermal toxicity had a better outcomes (HR for survival 0.42 (95% CI, 0.21–0.86) p of 0.01) [26]. The above-mentioned evidence prompted the opening of the randomized and controlled clinical trial phase III EXTREME, conducted by Vermorken et al., which aimed to evaluate the efficacy and safety of the combination of Cisplatin/Carboplatin +5FU + Cetuximab, in the front line, in the R/M HNSCC [28]. This study enrolled and randomized 442 patients with histological confirmed R/M HNSCC, no previously treated with systemic therapy, except previous chemotherapy combined with radiotherapy in the curative setting completed at least 6 months before. More than two hundred patients entered the standard chemotherapy arm, which included three-week treatment cycles of Cisplatin or Carboplatin+5-FU. An equal size control group of patients were assigned to the experimental arm which included the same chemotherapy + cetuximab. The protocol included a maximum of six chemotherapy cycles; for patients in the Cetuximab arm who had at least a disease stability, maintenance therapy with only Cetuximab was continued, until radiological evidence of disease progression or unacceptable toxicity. EGFR expression was tested by immunohistochemistry in more than four hundred tumors; of these, 98% were positive for EGFR staining and more than 80% had at least 40% of cells positive for its expression. The median duration of treatment with cetuximab was 18 weeks and 100 patients received maintenance therapy with anti-EGFR, for a median duration of 11 weeks. Chemotherapy compliance was similar between the two arms, suggesting that the addition of cetuximab does not affect tolerability to standard treatment. As for the evidence of efficacy, the median OS in the arm treated with chemotherapy alone was 7.4 months, compared to 10.1 months of the experimental arm (HR 0.80; 95% CI, 0.64–0.99; $p = 0.04$). Median PFS was 3.3 months in the control arm and 5.6 months in the experimental arm, showing a significant increase (HR 0.54; 95% CI, 0.43–0.67; $p < 0.001$). Among patients who continued the maintenance regimen with cetuximab, median PFS was 12 weeks from the start of maintenance therapy. The addition of cetuximab also resulted in a significant improvement in disease control rate and objective response, reaching an ORR of 36% and significantly increased compared to the 20% ORR shown by the chemotherapy regimen ($p < 0.001$). There was no significant difference between the two arms in terms of duration of response. The analysis of the safety profile showed a higher incidence of septic events, dermal toxicity, allergic infusion reactions and hypomagnesemia in patients treated with cetuximab. However, there was no significant increase in grade 3 or 4 adverse events in the cetuximab arm compared to the chemotherapy arm. The toxicity that led to discontinuation of treatment affected about 20% of patients in each arm. No correlation was observed between the degree of EGFR expression and the response rate in the two arms of the study, supporting the irrelevance of this parameter in predicting the response to Cetuximab [29].

In conclusion, the combination of Cisplatin/Carboplatin +5-FU + Cetuximab (EXTREME protocol) is an effective first line treatment for platinum sensitive R/M HNSCC, because it showed a gain in terms of overall survival. The clinical relevance of this evidence was remarkable, considering that since the introduction of cisplatin chemotherapy for R/M HNSCC, no combination regimen had brought significant improvements in overall survival [28].

4. No inferiority of the TPEx regimen compared to EXTREME

Evidence of the benefits in efficacy and antitumoral activity brought by the addition of cetuximab to standard chemotherapy protocols for relapse and/or metastatic platinum-sensitive tumors, laid to investigate the combination of Cetuximab to platinum and taxane-based chemotherapy. This protocol was evaluated in two consecutive phase II studies; the first (GORTEC 2008–2103 TPEx), a single arm study, was intended to explore its efficacy and tolerability while, in the subsequent trial (TPExtreme), the objective was to compare efficacy and the safety of this association with the combination of platinum +5-FU + Cetuximab [30, 31].

GORTEC 2008–2103 TPEx was conducted by Guigay et al. and the results were published in 2015, the primary objective was to evaluate the ORR while the secondary endpoints were PFS, OS and safety of the association regime. The study protocol was to run 4 cycles of the combination therapy, followed by maintenance with cetuximab only. Fifty-four patients with RM HNSCC, all with optimal performance status (ECOG PS 0-1) and less than 71 years old were enrolled to receive the treatment scheme. The results showed a significant antitumor activity of TPEx, with an ORR that reached 44.4%. The efficacy data were also encouraging, with a median PFS of 6.2 months and a median overall survival of 14 months, which increased to 7.1 and 16.8 months, respectively, in the population that had reached a disease control (SD, PR or CR) at the end of the 4 cycles of the TPEx protocol. The most common grade 3 or 4 adverse events were rash and non-febrile neutropenia. The safety profile was largely manageable and only in a few cases did therapeutic decreases or treatment discontinuations occurred.

To make more meaningful the comparison between the standard of care regimen EXTREME and the promising results of TPEx in terms of efficacy and antitumoral activity, Guigay et al. have started the multicenter and randomized clinical trial phase II GORTEC 2014–2101 TPExtreme [30]. The study aimed to compare the efficacy and safety of the TPEx regimen with the EXTREME protocol, as a therapeutic line for recurrent and/or metastatic tumors of the head-neck district, sensitive to platinum. The primary objective was to assess whether the TPEx protocol guaranteed a higher overall survival than the EXTREME standard of care. Involving 68 European centers, 541 patients were enrolled between 2014 and 2017, randomized with a ratio of 1:1 to the two treatment arms. Two-hundred and seventy patients were treated with the TPEx regimen for 4 cycles of therapy followed by maintenance with cetuximab and 270 patients were randomized to receive the EXTREME protocol, for 6 cycles and followed by maintenance with weekly Cetuximab. The median OS associated with TPEx was 14.5 months and 13.4 months for EXTREME, without evidence of significant difference between the two treatment protocols (HR 0.89; 95% CI, 0.74–1.08). Safety results suggested similar tolerability between the two regimens, 81% of patients treated with TPEx experienced grade 3 or 4 adverse events and 45% of patients had at least one serious adverse event; in patients treated with EXTREME, however, these percentages were 93 and 54%, respectively. In conclusion, although this clinical trial did not achieve its primary objective, as the overall survival of the two regimens was similar and without significant superiority of TPEx, the combination cisplatin

+ docetaxel + cetuximab showed a favorable safety profile. The evidence supported the adoption of TPEx as an alternative to the EXTREME therapeutic standard for platinum-sensitive R/M HNSCC.

5. CheckMate 141 introduces nivolumab for R/M HNSCC platinum-resistant

Both of the standard treatment alternatives in first line, EXTREME and TPEx, include chemotherapy with cisplatin/carboplatin and thus demonstrate their anti-tumor activity and efficacy on the platinum-sensitive diseases. Instead, the horizon of therapeutic possibilities for tumors that acquired resistance to platin was limited to the previously mentioned chemotherapeutic regimens, administered as single agents: Docetaxel, Paclitaxel, Methotrexate, Capecitabine. Previous work by Vermorken et al. on the activity of cetuximab as a single agent for platinum-resistant R/M HNSCC, supported the integration of this monoclonal antibody, either in monotherapy or in combination with the above chemotherapeutic agents, as a treatment option for patients experiencing disease progression to standard platinum-based regimens [25]. However, in the context of this therapeutic landscape of second line, lacking a well-established standard of care, the data on tumor response and overall survival were not encouraging, with an ORR ranging between 6 and 13% and a median OS of 3–6 months. With this background, the phase III CheckMake 141 trial compared the standard of care to nivolumab. This is an antibody agent capable of inhibiting, by binding and blocking PD-1, the immune checkpoint phase (immunecheckpoint-inhibitors - ICI) which is an important trick used by cancer cells to evade the immune system. Relapse and metastasis of HNSCC are favored by the phenomena of immune evasion, often mediated by the tumor expression of programmed death ligands (PD-L1 and PD-L2) interacting with the suppressive receptor PD-1 place on the immune system cells [32]. The CheckMate 141 study included recurrent and/or metastatic cancers of the oral cavity, larynx and pharynx that were no longer eligible for curative treatment and had progressed on or within 6 months of the last systemic platinum therapy.

There were 361 patients randomized with a 2:1 ratio to receive nivolumab or standard single agent chemotherapy. The primary objective was OS and secondary endpoints were ORR, PFS, the safety profile and implications for patients' quality of life. The control arm, consisting of 121 patients, was treated with weekly intravenous infusion of standard monotherapy based on cetuximab or methotrexate or docetaxel, chosen at the discretion of the oncologist, also based on any previous administration of cetuximab in the radical healing context or in the palliative regimens EXTREME/TPEx. Efficacy data showed that nivolumab resulted in a significant increase in overall survival and a 30% reduction in the risk of death compared to all single-agent therapeutic alternatives (HR 0.70; IC 97.73%, 0.51–0.96, p = 0.01). The median OS associated with immunotherapy was 7.5 months compared to 5.1 months of the control group (**Figure 1**). In particular, the efficacy parameters for each standard chemotherapy given in monotherapy, the median OS associated with cetuximab was 4.1 months (HR 0.47; 95% CI, 0.22–1.01), that associated with methotrexate 4.6 months (HR 0.64; 95% CI, 0.43–0.96) and that of patients treated with docetaxel at 5.8 months (HR 0.82; 95% CI, 0.53–1.28). The ORR of the arm in treatment with nivolumab was 13.3% compared to 5.8% found in patients under standard chemotherapy; the administration of anti-PD1 determined 6 complete and 26 partial responses.

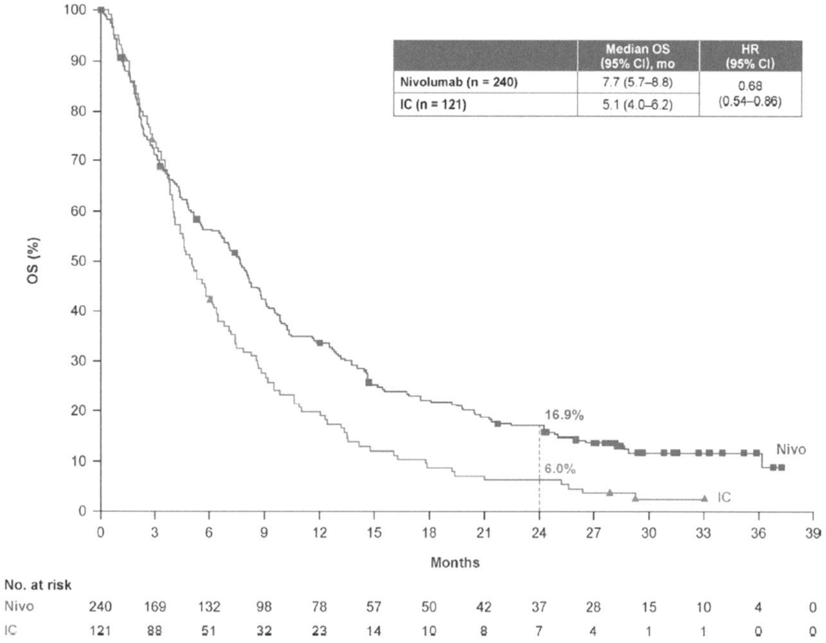

Figure 1.
Overall survival (OS) with a minimum follow-up of 24.2 months (intent-to-treat population) (treated by Ferris et al. [33]).

There was no significant difference between the two treatment groups in terms of PFS. Median PFS associated with nivolumab was 2 months, while that associated with standard monotherapy was 2.3 months.

In terms of safety data, the rate of adverse events was similar in both arms of the study with, however, a smaller number of toxicity grade 3 or 4 among patients treated with immunotherapy. Nivolumab was typically associated with fatigue, nausea, skin rash, inappetence and itching.

The results of CheckMate 141, published in 2016, represented a breakthrough in the treatment of this group of patients with a very poor prognosis, laying nivolumab to a standard of care for platinum resistant R/M HNSCC [32]. The phase III Keynote-040 trial compared pembrolizumab with established monotherapy as a standard of care [34]. Results were in line with that reported by Checkmate 141, supporting the significant superiority of immunotherapy, in terms of OS, compared to the standard regime of care with single agents. Between 2014 and 2016, 495 patients with recurrent and/or metastatic head-neck tumors that met the criteria of platinum-resistant were enrolled. Median OS in the immunotherapy arm was 8.4 months, significantly higher than that in the standard treatment arm, which was 6.9 months (HR 0.80; 95% CI, 0.65–0.98, $p = 0.0161$). In terms of antitumor activity, the objective response rate was 14.6% in patients treated with pembrolizumab and 10.1% in patients treated with single agents. Also relevant is the different median duration of response in the two arms, consistent with the results of Checkmate 141, it was 18.4 months in the immunotherapy group and 5 months in the standard therapy group. It should be noted that, stratifying the pembrolizumab group for PD-L1 expression, the fraction of patients who achieved a complete or partial response was higher among those with PD-L1 positivity. Also in Keynote-040 there was no significant difference in terms of progression-free survival between the two treatment arms.

The overall survival and safety profile results therefore support the clinical benefit of pembrolizumab in patients with platinum-resistant R/M HNSCC and justify future trials, either in monotherapy or combination regimens, for earlier stages of disease [34]. The relevance of the evidence from CheckMate 141 and Keynote-040 allowed to consolidate immunotherapy, with Nivolumab or Pembrolizumab as the first therapeutic option to be preferred, for patients with R/M HNSCC that has progressed in the context of treatment regimens containing cisplatin or carboplatin. Immunotherapy has shown superiority over standard single agent treatment, in terms of both anticancer activity and efficacy. It is important to note that the positivity at PD-L1 expression by the tumor and its microenvironment, identified by the combined positive score CPS, acts as a predictive biomarker for a better response to immunotherapy in R/M HNSCC.

6. Immunotherapy, alone or in combination with chemotherapy, becomes standard of care in I line for R/M HNSCC platinum sensitive

Pembrolizumab, associated with chemotherapy, represented a reasonable combination regime in HNSCC. On the one hand, cytotoxic drugs act by subverting the architecture of the tumor, which facilitates the expansion of the lymphocyte infiltrate in tumor micro-environment. On the other hand, these destructive effects result in the release of new tumor antigens and MHC expression, useful to mount a specific immune response against the disease. In addition, chemotherapy is able to eliminate myeloid suppressor cells and regulatory T lymphocytes, in favor of the accumulation of CD4+ T lymphocytes in the tumor microenvironment.

The phase III randomized clinical trial, Keynote-048 starts when the treatment scenario of first line for platinum-sensitive HNSCC had been widely established with the combination of chemotherapy and cetuximab in the EXTREME and TPEx protocols. Keynote-048 was an extremely important clinical study, as its evidence supported anti-PD-1 immunotherapy as a standard of care in this setting. The aim of the study was to determine whether pembrolizumab, as a single therapy or in combination with chemotherapy, improved OS compared to the standard chemotherapy. From two hundred centers in thirty-seven countries, 882 patients with R/M HNSCC platinum-naïve or not yet treated in the context of relapse and/or metastatic were enrolled. Before randomization, patients were stratified based on the CPS exhibited by the tumor and its microenvironment, identifying diseases with CPS 1 and diseases with CPS 20, although positivity to PD-L1 was not a necessary criterion for inclusion in the study. 85% of participants had a CPS greater than or equal to 1, while 43% had a CPS greater than or equal to 20. A second stratification was the HPV status for oropharyngeal tumors, which were determined by positivity for p16INK4A. Progression-free and overall survival of enrolled patients were the primary endpoints of this clinical trial. Secondly, the objective response rate in the three treatment arms was investigated, as well as the safety and tolerability of regimens including immunotherapy. Pembrolizumab, alone or in combination with chemotherapy, was hypothesized to be superior to the standard regimen of cetuximab + cisplatin/carboplatin +5-FU in terms of OS and PFS in patients with CPS 1, CPS 20 and in the total population enrolled. In addition, it was assumed that Pembrolizumab, alone or in combination with chemotherapy, was not inferior to the EXTREME protocol, also in terms of OS and PFS, in the total population studied.

In the second interim analysis, pembrolizumab monotherapy significantly increased OS compared to the standard chemotherapy arm alone, both in patients with CPS 20 (where, respectively, the median OS was 14.9 vs. 10.7 months, HR 0.77; IC 95%, 0.45–0.83; $p = 0.0007$), both in the group with CPS 1 (median OS of 12.3 months vs. 10.3 months, HR 0.78; IC 95%, 0.64–0.96; $p = 0.0086$). Pembrolizumab monotherapy was also not inferior to cetuximab + cisplatin/carboplatin +5-FU, considering the entire population studied (median OS respectively 11.6 vs. 10.7 months, HR 0.85; 95% CI, 0.71–1.03).

The combination of pembrolizumab + cisplatin/carboplatin +5-FU significantly increased overall survival compared to the standard regime of care: during the first interim analyses, this benefit was immediately evident for the total population (respectively, the median OS was 13 vs. 10.7 months, HR 0.77; 95% CI, 0.63–0.93, $p = 0.0034$). Subsequently, in the final analysis, the significant advantage of pembrolizumab associated with chemotherapy, compared to cetuximab + cisplatin/carboplatin +5-FU, also emerged in the stratified subgroups for CPS. In patients with CPS 20 the median OS was 14.7 versus 11 months respectively (HR 0.60; 95% CI, 0.45–0.82, $p = 0.0004$), while in patients with CPS 1 it was 13.6 vs. 10.4 months (HR 0.65; 95% CI, 0.53–0.80, $p < 0.0001$). Compared to the EXTREME protocol, monotherapy with pembrolizumab leads to a significant increase in overall survival, in tumors exhibiting CPS 20 and CPS 1. On the other hand, it is not less effective when considering the total population, not stratified for the degree of expression of PD-L1. When compared to the Cetuximab + platinum +5-FU regimen, pembrolizumab in combination with chemotherapy significantly prolongs overall survival of both CPS 20 and CPS 1 subgroups as well as the entire study population (**Figures 2** and **3**). Regarding progression-free survival and objective response rate, pembrolizumab, neither in monotherapy nor associated with chemotherapy, has provided significantly greater benefits than chemotherapy alone. The results of intermediate efficacy and antitumor activity were similar in all three treatments arms. Although the ORR under immunotherapy was not higher than that of the group treated with chemotherapy, at the final analysis of the antitumor parameters, the percentage of participants who had achieved an objective response, in the treatment arms with pembrolizumab + chemotherapy and with cetuximab + platinum +5-FU, was reported to stratification for CPS. In the subgroup with CPS ≥ 20, the ORR of the two arms was 43 and 38%, respectively; in patients with CPS ≥ 1, it was 36% in both treatment groups. Considering the total population, regardless of the expression of PD-L1, the ORR still reached 36%, both in the arm treated with immunotherapy + chemotherapy and in the group treated with cetuximab + chemotherapy. It should be pointed out, however, that the arms treated with immunotherapy had a higher number of complete responses. The duration of response was 16 months in the pembrolizumab arm and 2.5 months in the pembrolizumab + chemotherapy arm [36].

About the safety profile of Keynote 048, 55% of patients treated with pembrolizumab monotherapy experienced grade 3 or higher adverse effects, 83% treated with the combination of immunotherapy and chemotherapy and 83% of patients in the standard arm. Pembrolizumab does not exacerbate the toxicity associated with chemotherapy treatment, and vice versa.

The conclusions drawn from Keynote-048 represented a turning point in the therapeutic protocol of R/M HNSCC, changing the I line treatment [36]. The Food

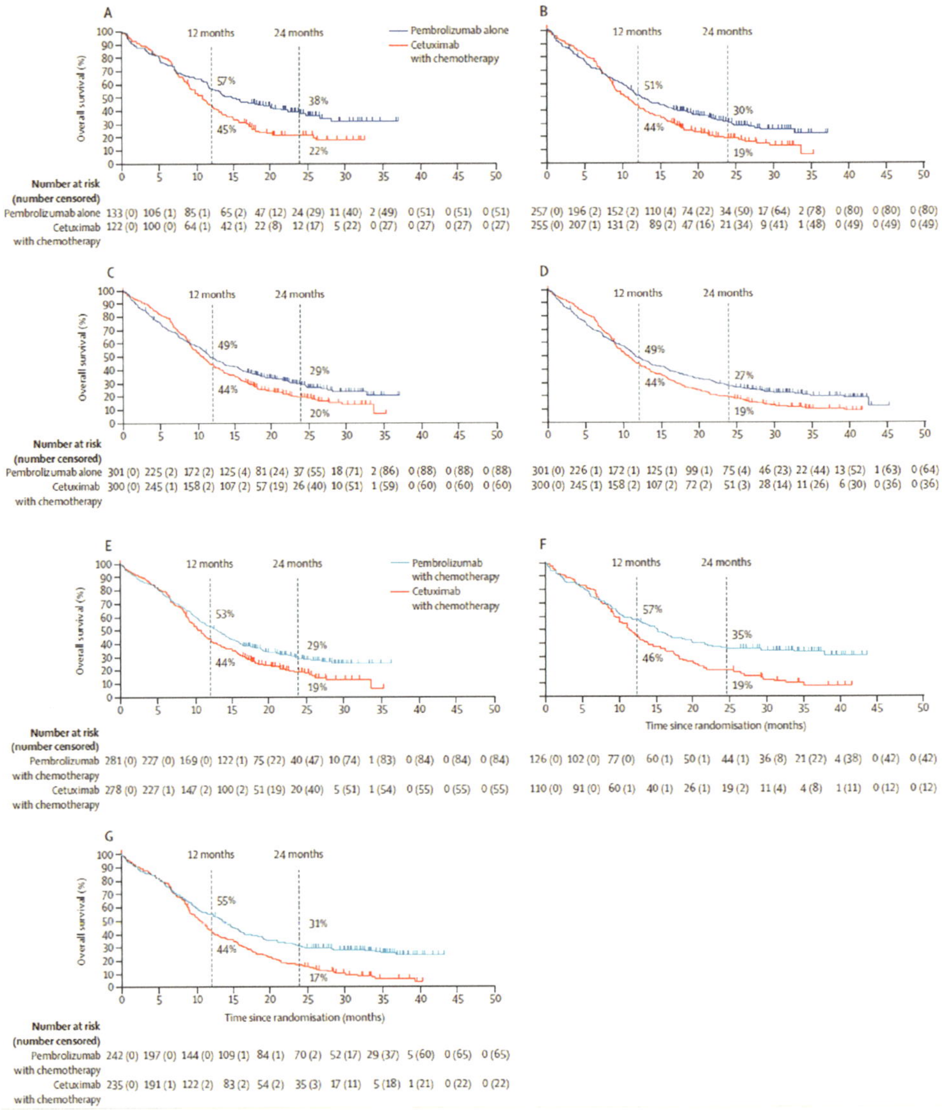

Figure 2.
Kaplan-Meier estimates of OS from Keynote 048 (Treated by Burtness et al. KEYNOTE-048 Investigators [35]).

and Drug Administration (FDA) has approved pembrolizumab in combination with chemotherapy as an I line of treatment for R/M HNSCC, regardless of the expression of PD-L; the indication of pembrolizumab in monotherapy was instead intended for cancers with CPS 1. The European Medicines Agency (EMA) has restricted the use of Pembrolizumab, either alone or in combination with chemotherapy, to patients with CPS 1, due to evidence that the increasing expression of PD-L1 correlates with a higher clinical benefit associated with pembrolizumab.

The indications that guide clinical practice for the treatment of R/M HNSCC cannot be separated from considering also other relevant aspects of the tumor, such as its

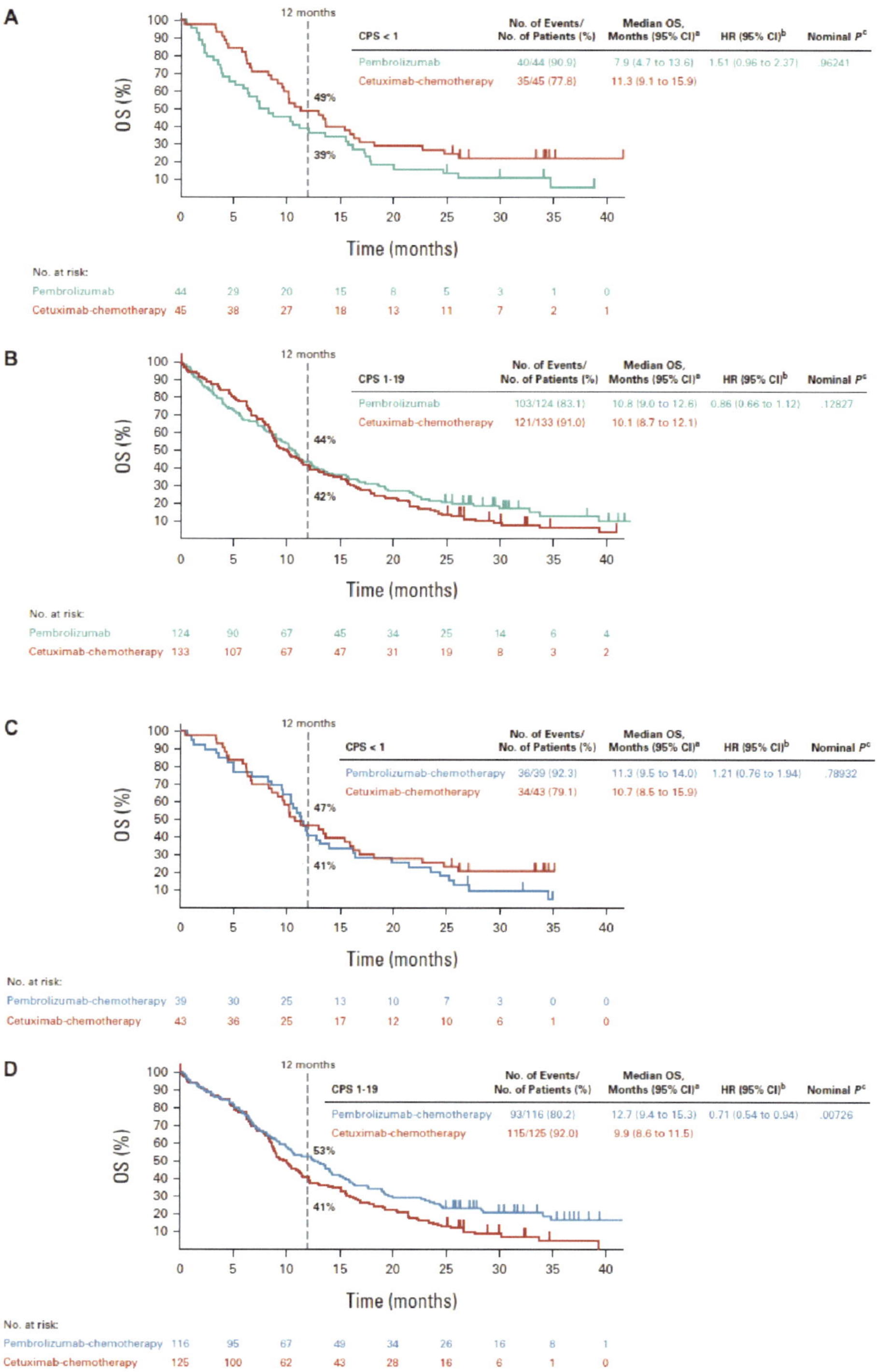

Figure 3.
Kaplan-Meier estimates of OS from Keynote 048 divided by CPS PD-L1 (treated from Burtness et al. [35]).

site, the burden of disease, and symptoms. These must contribute, together with the degree of expression of PD-L1, to the determination of the most suitable therapeutic protocol for the individual patient.

In conclusion, Pembrolizumab alone or combined with platinum and 5-FU represents the most appropriate line treatment for R/M HNSCC with CPS > = 1, while the EXTREME/TPEX protocol remains the standard for R/M HNSCC with CPS < 1. Pembrolizumab in combination with chemotherapy than monotherapy is preferred for patients with significant disease load, for tumors that manifest themselves as signs or symptoms and for tumor localization close to noble structures. For the clinical management of these cases, it is of primary importance to address the purpose of the treatment to obtain a tumor response that allows a reduction in size.

A further investigation, in the context of treatment with pembrolizumab combined with chemotherapy, was conducted by the clinical trial Keynote-B10 [35]. This is a single-arm phase IV study, which from 2020 to 2022 aimed to evaluate the activity and safety of pembrolizumab + carboplatin + paclitaxel as a combination of first line for platinum sensitive R/M HNSCC. The need to assess the clinical activity and tolerability of this regimen was based on evidence that 5-FU, as part of the standard protocol of chemotherapy combined with immunotherapy, was associated with some potential problems. The mode of administration, with daily intravenous infusions for four consecutive days and the toxicity profile with cardiac and gastrointestinal tropism contributed to the clinical need to research an alternative chemotherapy drug. The primary objective of this clinical trial was to evaluate the tolerability and objective response rate, in accordance with RECIST v1.1 criteria, for the combination regimen pembrolizumab + carboplatin + paclitaxel. One hundred and forty-nine patients with histological confirmation of R/M HNSCC were enrolled. At the final analysis of antitumor activity data, 49% of patients had achieved an objective tumor response, with seven patients who met a complete response. It is important to note that patients negative for PD-L1 expression (with CPS < 1) had an ORR of 65%, suggesting that this therapeutic combination is active regardless of the status of PD-L1. The median response time was 5.5 months, with 21% of objective responses lasting more than a year. Median overall survival was 13.1 months. In summary, pembrolizumab in combination with paclitaxel and carboplatin showed long-term anti-tumor activity and efficacy comparable to other established line regimens for these patients. The safety profile was manageable and tolerable, in line with previous studies investigating combination regimens containing paclitaxel [11]. The results of the Keynote-B10 study support the use of this treatment protocol as an additional line treatment option in patients with platinum-sensitive R/M HNSCC, regardless of PD-L1 expression.

The substantial benefits in terms of overall survival are influenced by a prolonged maintenance over time of the tumor responses associated with immunotherapy and raise the possibility that an early exposure to pembrolizumab can cause lasting alterations in the tumor microenvironment. The awakening of an antitumor immune response that is maintained over time affects the natural history of the tumor and sensitizes it to subsequent therapies, allowing a higher ORR to be obtained in systemic regimens following progression to immunotherapy [37]. The impact on survival of ICI is attributable not only to their direct anti-tumor effect, but also to the enhancement of the efficacy of chemotherapy in subsequent lines. It follows that the time to the second objective progression of disease can be extended by a rescue chemotherapy, following the failure of immunotherapy [38]. In a retrospective study, which aimed to investigate the effectiveness of chemotherapy after failure of the immunotherapy protocol, Saleh et al. highlighted that stabilization or objective disease response to previous immunotherapy was a predictor of better PFS and OS in patients who were then treated with salvage systemic therapy [37].

7. The therapeutic overview following progression to immunotherapy

The advent of immune checkpoint changed the treatment protocols for R/M HNSCC. The algorithm guiding the therapeutic approach makes a first distinction between disease sensitive or resistant to platinum-based chemotherapy. For patients refractory to platinum, never previously treated in the context of relapse and/or metastatic disease, only one therapeutic line has been defined, represented by nivolumab [32]. The relapse and/or metastatic disease, which is a candidate for systemic therapy with platinum is with pembrolizumab or cetuximab (EXTREME or TPEx). The most appropriate first intention option is chosen on the basis of the criteria described above, represented by the CPS presented and the patients and disease charcteristics.

Immunotherapy, which allows the restoration of co-stimulatory interactions on the effector cells of the immunity, follows the cytotoxic chemotherapy that increases the antigenic potential of the tumor. When the patient experiences disease progression to platinum and immunotherapy with nivolumab or pembrolizumab, the treatment options that can be pursued are no longer delineated by established therapeutic protocols. At this point in the patient's care path, treatment, either alone or in combination, with cetuximab and chemotherapy drugs such as taxane, capecitabine and methotrexate is again taking place, in the absence of unequivocal evidence identifying a clearly superior therapeutic regimen. Taking up what was stated at the beginning of this chapter, with the adoption of the established therapeutic algorithm as a standard of care and resorting to systemic treatments of rescue feasible for the patient, the platinum-sensitive disease reaches a median OS of 12–18 months, while patients refractory to platinum are burdened with worse prognosis, with a median OS of 8 months. Patients who cannot access any rescue protocol after immunotherapy failure have an even worse prognosis, with a median OS of only 3 months [38].

The evidence that emerged with Keynote-048 has exerted a profound influence on this still undefined therapeutic landscape. It has been found that even when the disease progression during immunotherapy, the anti-cancer effects of PD-1/PD-L1 inhibitors continue to persist over time and may enhance the effects of subsequent chemotherapy. The hypothesis that previous treatment with ICI could increase the efficacy of subsequent chemotherapy has prompted research to experiment with chemotherapy regimens and molecular target therapies. Several studies have been carried out to investigate which monotherapy or combined regimen could maximize its potential activity, taking advantage of the long-term benefits guaranteed by the previous immunotherapy. In this context, the publication of Saleh et al. from 2019 will be given priority attention [37]. This is a retrospective study that analyzed data from four French centers between 2014 and 2018 concerning the clinical activity of rescue treatments administered after progression to ICI in patients with R/M HNSCC. The study was initiated on the basis of the results from the Keynote-048 trial, which, in turn, were consistent with evidence in the context lung carcinomas, of an increase in tumor response to SCT after progression to immunotherapy. Initiated to study the reproducibility of the phenomenon also in recurrent and/or metastatic head-neck tumors, this retrospective study reported an objective response rate of 30%, to support the effective potential synergy between immunotherapy followed by systemic rescue therapy. Data from 82 patients were analyzed, whose median age at the onset of therapy was 60 years. The median interval between the last dose of immune-checkpoint inhibitors and the start of salvage chemotherapy was 1 month. For systemic regimens administered after progression to immunotherapy, 56% of the patients analyzed received a taxane-based therapy. Of these, 26 patients were treated with paclitaxel or docetaxel alone, 17 patients with cetuximab + platinum+taxane and 3 patients with taxane + platinum. 37% of patients received a systemic regimen containing platinum, 16 patients were treated with the combination of platinum +5-FU + Cetuximab, 3 patients with 8 patients with Carboplatino + Cetuximab and 3 patients with Carboplatino + Paclitaxel. Activity and efficacy data revealed that the ORR to salvage chemotherapy was 30%, with 3 complete responses and 22 partial responses. The disease control rate reached 57%. The combination of cetuximab + platinum+taxane was the rescue regimen with the highest number of objective responses. Median OS was 7.8 months, while the median PFS was 3.6 months. Multivariate analysis identified that the type of systemic regimen received before immunotherapy and the best response to ICI represent the two main predictors for the OS in this group of patients.

After previous line of ICI, the rate of objective response shown to rescue chemotherapy is significantly higher than what was recorded, before the advent of immunotherapy for R/M HNSCC [25]. This finding again highlights the long-term, natural history implications of the disease, which had the introduction of immunotherapy as a standard treatment protocol for recurrent and/or metastatic head-neck cancers. In 2021, Pestana et al. pubblished a retrospective study on this topic [39]. The clinical data of 43 patients were analyzed, in 58% of the sample, immunotherapy had been administered as the first line of treatment and more than 90% of the patients had been exposed to platinum-containing chemotherapy regimens. After progression to immunotherapy, 37% of patients received Cetuximab as a single agent, 32% were treated with chemotherapy drugs in monotherapy, 18% with a combination of chemotherapy and Cetuximab, while 11% of the sample received chemotherapy in combination with other experimental drugs. The objective response rate achieved with systemic rescue therapy, administered after immunotherapy failure, was 43% and median overall survival of 8.4 months. These results were significantly better than those obtained before the introduction of R/M HNSCC immunotherapy with systemic therapies of line II and subsequent lines. A specific focus on the clinical benefit associated with Cetuximab was given by the study conducted by Cabezas-Camarero et al., which retrospectively investigated the safety and efficacy of Cetuximab salvage chemotherapy, as a treatment line following immunotherapy [40]. Twenty three patients with R/M HNSCC who had shown disease progression to standard of care with ICI were included. Most of the sample had significant comorbidities, a compromised performance status and a substantial disease burden. About half of the patients had already received a systemic therapy line prior to the immunotherapeutic protocol. The rescue treatment consisted of Cetuximab combined with weekly Paclitaxel (ERBITAX protocol), with Carboplatin + Paclitaxel weekly (CARBITAX protocol), with 5-FU + Cisplatin trisettimanals (EXTREME protocol) or with Cisplatin (wkCDDP-Cetuximab protocol). In the whole sample, Cetuximab salvage chemotherapy resulted in an objective response rate of 56.5%, with 2 complete responses and 11 partial responses. The disease control rate reached 78.3%, associated with a median reduction in tumor volume of 57% among patients who had exhibited an objective response. Ten patients had received systemic treatment before immunotherapy, typically with combination regimens containing Cetuximab, platinum and taxanes or 5-FU, during which they had an objective response rate of 40%. In this subgroup of patients, the ORR at rescue therapy reached 60%. Median overall survival was 12 months, progression-free survival was 6 months. The lifesaving regimen with the highest number of objective responses was cetuximab in combination with paclitaxel weekly (ERBITAX). The study showed that Cetuximab-based salvage chemotherapy, given after immunotherapy failure, could be highly effective even in fragile and multi-treated patients.

Finally, it is appropriate to report the data from Interlink-1, a phase III study closed for futility which, however, represents an interesting starting point for the purposes of this paper [41]. This is a multicenter, randomized, double-blind and placebo-controlled study, always conducted in the context of resistance to immunotherapy, which aimed to compare Cetuximab + placebo with Cetuximab + Monalizumab. The latter is a monoclonal antibody, with immunostimulating properties, which acts by blocking the immune checkpoint between MHC-I, on cancer cells, and NKG2A, an inhibitory receptor placed on NK cells. Preliminary data suggested that the combination of cetuximab and monalizumab could express anti-tumor activity of clinical utility. In a 2:1 ratio, 480 patients were randomized in the two treatment arms to make up the global population. The study sample was also stratified according to HPV status. The primary population for analysis was the subgroup with disease not related to HPV. The primary endpoint was OS in the HPV negative group. The secondary targets were global population OS, PFS, ORR, duration of response; these endpoints were evaluated in both the non-HPV reported subgroup and in whole population. Median overall survival was 8.8 months in the Monalizumab + Cetuximab arm and 8.6 months in the placebo + Cetuximab receiving arm (HR 1.00; 95% CI, 0.66–1.54). The criteria for interruption for futility have been met. The median PFS in the arms Monalizumab + Cetuximab and placebo + Cetuximab was 3.6 and 3.8 months respectively (HR 1.11; 95% CI, 0.79–1.57). The ORR in the group receiving Monalizumab + Cetuximab was 15.2% while that of the arm treated with only Cetuximab was 23.9%; the median DORs were 5.7 and 5.6 months, respectively. The median OS in participants who received immunotherapy immediately prior to randomization was 9.1 months compared with 7.4 months for patients who did not receive the immediate pre-enrollment (HR 0.85; 95% IC, 0.56–1.30). The efficacy of Monalizumab + Cetuximab compared to Cetuximab alone was similar, regardless of whether participants had received immunotherapy prior to this treatment protocol. Similar results were observed in the whole population for all efficacy endpoints; safety profiles were found to be similar between the two treatment arms. In this population of patients with R/M HNSCC, previously treated with platinum-based chemotherapy and an immune checkpoint inhibitor, the combination of Monalizumab and Cetuximab did not improve overall survival, compared to monotherapy with cetuximab. Failure to reach the primary endpoint meant that the clinical trial was terminated for reasons of futility. Neither the secondary efficacy and activity endpoints showed improvement from the addition of Monalizumab to Cetuximab. In particular, the ORR in the arm treated with Cetuximab as a single agent, 23.9%, was higher than expected based on the studies mentioned above, who investigated the activity of cetuximab in monotherapy as a treatment line following failure of the standard of care. Based on the evidence until the start of Interlink-1, treatment with cetuximab after disease progression to platinum-based chemotherapy resulted in an ORR range of 6–13%. As reported on several occasions in this paragraph, the high response rate to treatment with Cetuximab alone could be described in light of the long-term anti-tumor effect that ICI drugs have on the immune system, resulting in an increase in effectiveness and activity for systemic therapies that are administered subsequently. The ORR in participants with HPV-positive oropharyngeal carcinoma was poor; in both treatment arms, patients negative for HPV reached an ORR of 18.1%, while among 48 enrolled with HPV-related oropharyngeal carcinoma, only one objective response was observed. These results echo previous evidence suggesting limited or absent activity of cetuximab in HPV-positive HNSCC. This study is worthy of a mention in this treatise as it has provided, for the first time in the kaleidoscopic therapeutic landscape of R/M HNSCC resistant to immunotherapy, the anti-tumor activity data exclusively associated with treatment with Cetuximab as a single agent, in treatment lines following ICI.

8. Conclusion

From 1980 to the present, clinical research on HNSCC has produced evidence that has changed the approach, outcomes, and expectations of systemic medical treatments in RM HNSCC. Platinum-based chemotherapy is still a cornerstone in the treatment of these patients. Early phase III studies showed that cisplatin monotherapy was more effective than other chemotherapy drugs, and combination regimens, such as cisplatin +5-FU, showed a better ORR than cisplatin alone. Subsequently, a new step forward was made with the introduction of the first target therapy, cetuximab, which further improved survival rates with long progression-free intervals. The phase III study Chemate141 and then the Keynote048 study introduced ICIs into therapeutic drugs for these patients, changing their natural history and introducing new research insights. Despite this, long surviving patients are still few and there is still much to discover about the biology of the tumor.

Author details

Andrea Alberti
Medical Oncology Unit, Department of Medical and Surgical Specialties, Radiological Sciences, and Public Health, University of Brescia at the Azienda Socio Sanitaria Territoriale (ASST)-Spedali Civili, Brescia, Italy

*Address all correspondence to: a.alberti015@unibs.it

References

[1] Numeri I, Cancro D. Associazione italiana di oncologia medica (AIOM), I numeri del cancro in Italia. 2019. Available from: https://www.registri-tumori.it/cms/pubblicazioni/i-numeri-del-cancro-italia-2019

[2] Ghosh S, Shah PA, Johnson FM. Novel systemic treatment modalities including immunotherapy and molecular targeted therapy for recurrent and metastatic head and neck squamous cell carcinoma. International Journal of Molecular Sciences. 2022;**23**:7889

[3] Lee AW, Law SC, Foo W, Poon YF, Cheung FK, Chan DK, et al. Retrospective analysis of patients with nasopharyngeal carcinoma treated during 1976-1985: Survival after local recurrence. International Journal of Radiation Oncology, Biology, Physics. 1993;**26**:773-782

[4] Fakhry C, Zhang Q, Nguyen-Tan PF, Rosenthal D, El-Naggar A, Garden AS, et al. Human papillomavirus and overall survival after progression of oropharyngeal squamous cell carcinoma. Journal of Clinical Oncology. 2014;**32**:3365-3373

[5] Machiels J-P, René Leemans C, Golusinski W, Grau C, Licitra L, Gregoire V. Squamous cell carcinoma of the oral cavity, larynx, oropharynx and hypopharynx: EHNS–ESMO–ESTRO clinical practice guidelines for diagnosis, treatment and follow-up. Annals of Oncology. 2020;**31**:1462-1475

[6] Morton RP, Rugman F, Dorman EB, Stoney PJ, Wilson JA, McCormick M, et al. Cisplatinum and bleomycin for advanced or recurrent squamous cell carcinoma of the head and neck: A randomised factorial phase III controlled trial. Cancer Chemotherapy and Pharmacology. 1985;**15**(3):283-289. DOI: 10.1007/BF00263902

[7] A phase III randomised trial of cistplatinum, methotrextate, cisplatinum + methotrexate and cisplatinum + 5-FU in end stage squamous carcinoma of the head and neck. Liverpool Head and Neck Oncology Group. British Journal of Cancer. 1990;**61**:311-315

[8] Kish JA, Weaver A, Jacobs J, Cummings G, Al-Sarraf M. Cisplatin and 5-fluorouracil infusion in patients with recurrent and disseminated epidermoid cancer of the head and neck. Cancer. 1984;**53**:1819-1824

[9] Jacobs C, Lyman G, Velez-García E, Sridhar KS, Knight W, Hochster H, et al. A phase III randomized study comparing cisplatin and fluorouracil as single agents and in combination for advanced squamous cell carcinoma of the head and neck. Journal of Clinical Oncology. 1992;**10**:257-263

[10] Forastiere AA, Metch B, Schuller DE, Ensley JF, Hutchins LF, Triozzi P, et al. Randomized comparison of cisplatin plus fluorouracil and carboplatin plus fluorouracil versus methotrexate in advanced squamous-cell carcinoma of the head and neck: A southwest oncology group study. Journal of Clinical Oncology. 1992;**10**:1245-1251

[11] Gibson MK, Li Y, Murphy B, Hussain MHA, DeConti RC, Ensley J, et al. Randomized phase III evaluation of cisplatin plus fluorouracil versus cisplatin plus paclitaxel in advanced head and neck cancer (E1395): An intergroup trial of the eastern cooperative oncology group. Journal of Clinical Oncology. 2005;**23**:3562-3567

[12] Urba S, Van Herpen CML, Sahoo TP, Shin DM, Licitra L, Mezei K, et al. Pemetrexed in combination with cisplatin versus cisplatin monotherapy in patients with recurrent or metastatic head and neck cancer: Final results of a randomized, double-blind, placebo-controlled, phase 3 study. Cancer. 2012;**118**:4694-4705

[13] Price KAR, Cohen EE. Current treatment options for metastatic head and neck cancer. Current Treatment Options in Oncology. 2012;**13**:35-46

[14] Smith RE, Thornton DE, Allen J. A phase II trial of paclitaxel in squamous cell carcinoma of the head and neck with correlative laboratory studies. Seminars in Oncology. 1995;**22**:41-46

[15] Forastiere AA, Shank D, Neuberg D, Taylor SG, DeConti RC, Adams G. Final report of a phase II evaluation of paclitaxel in patients with advanced squamous cell carcinoma of the head and neck: An eastern cooperative oncology group trial (PA390). Cancer. 1998;**82**:2270-2274

[16] Dreyfuss AI, Clark JR, Norris CM, Rossi RM, Lucarini JW, Busse PM, et al. Docetaxel: An active drug for squamous cell carcinoma of the head and neck. Journal of Clinical Oncology. 1996;**14**:1672-1678

[17] Couteau C, Chouaki N, Leyvraz S, Oulid-Aissa D, Lebecq A, Domenge C, et al. A phase II study of docetaxel in patients with metastatic squamous cell carcinoma of the head and neck. British Journal of Cancer. 1999;**81**:457-462

[18] Catimel G, Verweij J, Mattijssen V, Hanauske A, Piccart M, Wanders J, et al. Docetaxel (Taxotere®): An active drug for the treatment of patients with advanced squamous cell carcinoma of the head and neck. Annals of Oncology. 1994;**5**:533-537

[19] On behalf of the Spanish Head and Neck Cancer Treatment Group (TTCC), Martinez-Trufero J, Isla D, Adansa JC, Irigoyen A, Hitt R, et al. Phase II study of capecitabine as palliative treatment for patients with recurrent and metastatic squamous head and neck cancer after previous platinum-based treatment. British Journal of Cancer. 2010;**102**:1687-1691

[20] Pivot X, Raymond E, Laguerre B, Degardin M, Cals L, Armand JP, et al. Pemetrexed disodium in recurrent locally advanced or metastatic squamous cell carcinoma of the head and neck. British Journal of Cancer. 2001;**85**:649-655

[21] Argiris A, Li Y, Murphy BA, Langer CJ, Forastiere AA. Outcome of elderly patients with recurrent or metastatic head and neck cancer treated with cisplatin-based chemotherapy. Journal of Clinical Oncology. 2004;**22**:262-268

[22] Kiyota N, Tahara M, Kadowaki S, Fuse N, Doi T, Minami H, et al. Systemic chemotherapy with cisplatin plus 5-FU (PF) for recurrent or metastatic squamous cell carcinoma of the head and neck (R/M SCCHN): Efficacy and safety of a lower dose of PF (80/800) at a single institution in Japan. Japanese Journal of Clinical Oncology. 2009;**39**:225-230

[23] Baselga J, Trigo JM, Bourhis J, Tortochaux J, Cortés-Funes H, Hitt R, et al. Phase II multicenter study of the antiepidermal growth factor receptor monoclonal antibody cetuximab in combination with platinum-based chemotherapy in patients with platinum-refractory metastatic and/or recurrent squamous cell carcinoma of the head and neck. Journal of Clinical Oncology. 2005;**23**:5568-5577

[24] Herbst RS, Arquette M, Shin DM, Dicke K, Vokes EE, Azarnia N, et al. Phase II multicenter study of the epidermal growth factor receptor antibody cetuximab and cisplatin for recurrent and refractory squamous cell carcinoma of the head and neck. Journal of Clinical Oncology. 2005;**23**:5578-5587

[25] Vermorken JB, Trigo J, Hitt R, Koralewski P, Diaz-Rubio E, Rolland F, et al. Open-label, uncontrolled, multicenter phase II study to evaluate the efficacy and toxicity of cetuximab as a single agent in patients with recurrent and/or metastatic squamous cell carcinoma of the head and neck who failed to respond to platinum-based therapy. Journal of Clinical Oncology. 2007;**25**:2171-2177

[26] Burtness B, Goldwasser MA, Flood W, Mattar B, Forastiere AA. Phase III randomized trial of cisplatin plus placebo compared with cisplatin plus cetuximab in metastatic/recurrent head and neck cancer: An eastern cooperative oncology group study. Journal of Clinical Oncology. 2005;**23**:8646-8654

[27] Bourhis J, Rivera F, Mesia R, Awada A, Geoffrois L, Borel C, et al. Phase I/II study of cetuximab in combination with cisplatin or carboplatin and fluorouracil in patients with recurrent or metastatic squamous cell carcinoma of the head and neck. Journal of Clinical Oncology. 2006;**24**:2866-2872

[28] Vermorken JB, Mesia R, Rivera F, Remenar E, Kawecki A, Rottey S, et al. Platinum-based chemotherapy plus cetuximab in head and neck cancer. The New England Journal of Medicine. 2008;**359**:1116-1127

[29] Bossi P, Resteghini C, Paielli N, Licitra L, Pilotti S, Perrone F. Prognostic and predictive value of EGFR in head and neck squamous cell carcinoma. Oncotarget. 2016;**7**:74362-74379

[30] Guigay J, Aupérin A, Fayette J, Saada-Bouzid E, Lafond C, Taberna M, et al. Cetuximab, docetaxel, and cisplatin versus platinum, fluorouracil, and cetuximab as first-line treatment in patients with recurrent or metastatic head and neck squamous-cell carcinoma (GORTEC 2014-01 TPExtreme): A multicentre, open-label, randomised, phase 2 trial. The Lancet Oncology. 2021;**22**:463-475

[31] Guigay J, Fayette J, Dillies AF, Sire C, Kerger JN, Tennevet I, et al. Cetuximab, docetaxel, and cisplatin as first-line treatment in patients with recurrent or metastatic head and neck squamous cell carcinoma: A multicenter, phase II GORTEC study. Annals of Oncology. 2015;**26**:1941-1947

[32] Ferris RL, Blumenschein G, Fayette J, Guigay J, Colevas AD, Licitra L, et al. Nivolumab for recurrent squamous-cell carcinoma of the head and neck. The New England Journal of Medicine. 2016;**375**:1856-1867

[33] Ferris RL et al. Nivolumab vs investigator's choice in recurrent or metastatic squamous cell carcinoma of the head and neck: 2-year long-term survival update of CheckMate 141 with analyses by tumor PD-L1 expression. Oral Oncology. 2018;**81**:45-51

[34] Cohen EEW, Soulières D, Le Tourneau C, Dinis J, Licitra L, Ahn M-J, et al. Pembrolizumab versus methotrexate, docetaxel, or cetuximab for recurrent or metastatic head-and-neck squamous cell carcinoma (KEYNOTE-040): A randomised, open-label, phase 3 study. The Lancet. 2019;**393**:156-167

[35] Dzienis M, Cundom J, Fuentes CS, Spreafico A, Nordlinger M, Pastor AV, et al. Pembrolizumab plus carboplatin and paclitaxel as first-line therapy

for recurrent/metastatic head and neck squamous cell carcinoma (KEYNOTE-B10): A single-arm phase IV trial. Journal of Clinical Oncology. 2024;**42**:2989-2999

[36] Burtness B, Harrington KJ, Greil R, Soulières D, Tahara M, De Castro G, et al. Pembrolizumab alone or with chemotherapy versus cetuximab with chemotherapy for recurrent or metastatic squamous cell carcinoma of the head and neck (KEYNOTE-048): A randomised, open-label, phase 3 study. The Lancet. 2019;**394**:1915-1928

[37] Saleh K, Daste A, Martin N, Pons-Tostivint E, Auperin A, Herrera-Gomez RG, et al. Response to salvage chemotherapy after progression on immune checkpoint inhibitors in patients with recurrent and/or metastatic squamous cell carcinoma of the head and neck. European Journal of Cancer. 2019;**121**:123-129

[38] Watanabe T, Oka H, Nagashima K, Nishi H, Kumai Y, Iijima H, et al. Clinical outcomes of recurrent or metastatic head and neck cancer after failure of platinum and nivolumab: A multicenter retrospective study. The Oncologist. 2025;**30**:oyaf018

[39] Pestana RC, Becnel M, Rubin ML, Torman DK, Crespo J, Phan J, et al. Response rates and survival to systemic therapy after immune checkpoint inhibitor failure in recurrent/metastatic head and neck squamous cell carcinoma. Oral Oncology. 2020;**101**:104523

[40] Cabezas-Camarero S, Cabrera-Martín MN, Merino-Menéndez S, Paz-Cabezas M, García-Barberán V, Sáiz-Pardo Sanz M, et al. Safety and efficacy of cetuximab-based salvage chemotherapy after checkpoint inhibitors in head and neck cancer. The Oncologist. 2021;**26**:e1018-e1035

[41] Fayette J, Licitra L, Harrington K, Haddad R, Siu LL, Liu Y-C, et al. INTERLINK-1: A phase III, randomized, placebo-controlled study of monalizumab plus cetuximab in recurrent/metastatic head and neck squamous cell carcinoma. Clinical Cancer Research. 1 Jul 2025;**31**(13):2617-2627